Coping
With
Cancer

John E. Packo

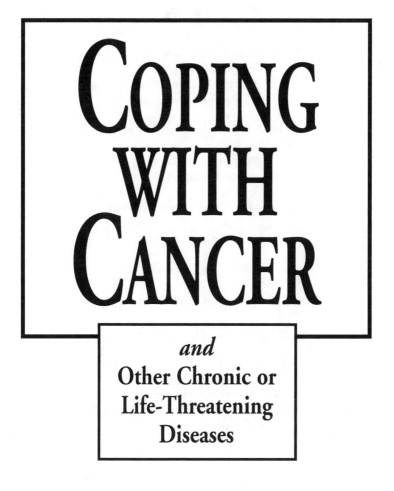

COPING WITH CANCER

and
Other Chronic or
Life-Threatening
Diseases

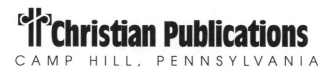

Christian Publications

CAMP HILL, PENNSYLVANIA

Christian Publications
3825 Hartzdale Drive
Camp Hill, PA 17011
www.cpi-horizon.com

Faithful, biblical publishing since 1883

Coping with Cancer
ISBN: 0-87509-438-4

LOC Catalog Card Number: 90-62157

© 1991 by Christian Publications, Inc.

Printed in the United States of America

99 00 01 02 03   7 6 5 4 3

Unless otherwise indicated, Scripture
taken from the Holy Bible:
New International Version ®.
© 1973, 1978, 1984 by the International Bible Society.
Used by permission of Zondervan Bible Publishers.

CONTENTS

PREFACE

Cancer, with over 200 disguises, has become an epidemic disease. The American Cancer Society estimates that nearly one in every three persons living today eventually will contract cancer. As a victim of advanced diffuse histiocytic lymphoma, I became one of those statistics.

It began when I struggled for three months with an energy-draining bronchial condition that caused endless coughing and gasping for air. When treatments by a local doctor were unsuccessful, I went to the University of Michigan Hospital. Following two weeks of tests, the oncologist confronted me with his diagnosis.

"You have diffuse histiocytic lymphoma in the advanced stage," the doctor announced. Privately to my wife he added, "If the chemotherapy doesn't work, he has one month to live."

Only one month for this fast-acting lymphoma to finish its deadly work! Was this really happening to me?

I was in a difficult situation. As a pastor, I had encouraged others to trust in the unlimited resources of God. That was my field of expertise. But now a new and unwanted experience faced me. Rather than being counselor, I was now victim. How would I handle this ex-

1

perience? Would I practice what I preached? Would I observe the disciplines and principles I had shared with others in their sicknesses? Would these measures work for *me*?

One year later I sat again with my oncologist. "Just this morning," he began, "during a conference on your case, a team of physicians looked over your medical records. We all came to the same conclusion: *You are a miracle.*"

Pastors ministering to cancer patients and many lay people with family members stricken by cancer have encouraged me to write a book that they could recommend. This is my attempt. I have written from a biblical viewpoint and from a pastor's heart, hoping to share what I have learned as I walked through the world of cancer.

I discovered that the main battlefield is internal—in our hearts. During this warfare, our inner person carries on a continuous conversation. I have coined the term "heart-talk" to describe it. In the struggle for wholeness, our heart-talk is either creative or noncreative. If we allow negative thinking and unhealthy emotions to control us in the daily conflicts, we are noncreative. However, if we permit biblical principles to fill us with positive thoughts and healthy emotions that result in spiritual victories, we are creative.

In what follows, I have presented 12 "creative choices" that took me through my fight against cancer. As I look back on the experience, I am overcome by a sense of wonder. I praise our good God. I feel like King David when he reminded Israel of God's marvelous deeds in their behalf:

> Look at the Lord and his strength;
>   seek his face always.
> Remember the wonders he has done.
>   (1 Chronicles 16:11–12)

John E. Packo
Cincinnati, Ohio
March, 1990

"I did not choose cancer but I choose to trust God for courage to cope with cancer."

Have I not commanded you? Be strong and courageous. Do not be terrified; do not be discouraged, for the Lord your God will be with you wherever you go. Joshua 1:9

History is a record of our decisions, good and bad. Our lives are the sum total of our decisions and their consequences.[1]
Vance Havner

If you were to visit our home, you would see a number of oil paintings on the walls. Although they are not Rembrandts or Monets, they are colorful and attractive. At least they are to me. I created them. And if you wanted to know when, I would reply, "The year I was treated for cancer."

The paintings are special to me because something creative and beautiful came out of the unpleasantness of cancer. I chose to be creative during that crisis. The paintings are a reminder of the power of choice, the gift of art and the Lord's healing power that gave me extended life to serve Him.

As far as I was concerned, giving up in a seemingly impossible situation was not the answer. I could have wallowed in self-pity, but I chose to pick up the brushes and create beautiful scenes on canvas. On blue skies I stroked bright sunshine that sent its warm rays past white puffy clouds to red and golden trees whose glorious colors were mirrored from peaceful lakes. With a song in my heart I would sing, "It is well, it is well with my soul."

As I painted and sang, the thoughts of cancer were replaced by creative thoughts of good things. The therapy assisted my body in the healing process.

The Bible encourages us to occupy our minds with that which is good and praiseworthy:

> Finally, brothers, whatever is true, whatever is noble, whatever is right, whatever is pure, whatever is lovely, whatever is admirable—if anything is excellent or praiseworthy—think about such things. (Philippians 4:8)

You may have no artistic bent. But you can be as creative as an artist when you choose to pick up the Bible and allow its message to paint the beauty of Christlikeness in your character.

One of the greatest wonders in life is the power of choice. God did not choose to create us as robots programmed to move at the push of a computer button. He created us in His image and gave us the creative capacity to make decisions. His divine intention is for us to choose to cooperate completely with Him. He gave us the freedom to determine how we will respond to the crisis of cancer, whether in our own life or in the lives of others.

Will it be creatively or otherwise?

The heart: center for choices

In the Museum of Science and Industry in Chicago is a gigantic replica of the human heart, large enough for visitors to go inside it and observe it in action. The valves and the other intricate parts are functioning. There is even the *thump, thump, thump* as it beats! As we know, the heart is a pump that pushes blood to all parts of the body. The blood leaves the heart by one channel and returns through another. This circulation of blood continues every moment of our lives.

As a physical organ, the heart is the center of strength and physical life. David expressed it this way:

> My heart pounds, my strength fails me;
>   even the light has gone from my eyes.
> (Psalm 38:10)

Figuratively, the heart is that hidden spring deep within us from which all of our behavior flows. It is the control center of the spiritual life. Conscious thinking, feeling and decision-making flow from this source. I have diagrammed it like this:

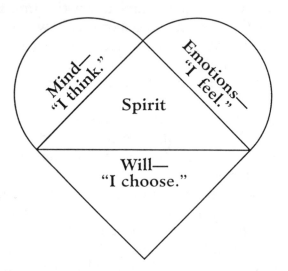

The heart is used as a figure of speech for the inner life in contrast to external appearance. God said to Samuel, "Man looks at the outward appearance, but the Lord looks at the heart" (1 Samuel 16:7c). Peter contrasts external adornment with "the hidden person of the heart, with the incorruptible ornament of a gentle and quiet spirit, which is very precious in the sight of God" (1 Peter 3:4 NKJ). God knows the motives behind our choices, and the Bible declares, "He will bring to light what is hidden in darkness and will expose the motives of men's hearts" (1 Corinthians 4:5b).

Heart-talk: our inner conversation

It is in this deep inner recess where we formulate choices as we continue to think and feel throughout the course of our actions. In this inner process we are using words to talk to ourselves about every daily experience of every waking moment. It is this internal relating that I have called "heart-talk." Notice these Bible verses:

> He has said in his heart, "I shall not be moved." (Psalm 10:6 NKJ)

> Now Hannah spoke in her heart . . . (1 Samuel 1:13 NKJ)

> And David said in his heart . . . (1 Samuel 27:1 NKJ)

Heart-talk is a continuous internal conversation that is influenced by our beliefs. It is essential, therefore, for our beliefs to be Bible-centered. Creative choices originate from correct biblical thinking that has been internalized in our own thinking. Jesus said, "You will know the truth, and the truth will set you free" (John 8:32). Freedom is not "doing our own thing"; it is choosing to be governed by the truth of God's Word. This delivers us from guilt, misery, worry and enslaving habits such as substance abuse and tobacco addiction (the leading cause of lung cancer). It frees us to have love, joy, peace, security, assurance and a clear conscience.

For the sake of health to the "whole body," a wise Father God instructs us to govern our hearts according to the truth of His Word:

> My son, pay attention to what I say;
>   listen closely to my words.
> Do not let them out of your sight,
>   keep them within your heart;
> for they are life to those who find them
>   and health to a man's whole body.
> Above all else, guard your heart,
>   for it is the wellspring of life.
>   (Proverbs 4:20–23)

I see in that instruction four guidelines to be observed by the person thrust into the world of cancer.

1. *Concentrate on the Word of God*—"Pay attention to what I say" (4:20). Elisabeth Kubler-Ross made famous a list of five psychological preparations for death. The five are (1) shock or denial, (2) anger, (3) bargaining with God ("I'll reform if You spare me"), (4) depression, (5) acceptance. The same five stages are also the common experience of cancer patients. Friends and loved ones may also go through them. Attentive listening to the Word of God

will reduce the stress as a person works through the five stages.

2. *Reflect on what God says*—"Do not let them out of your sight" (4:21). Bible meditation is an effective method of seeing and sensing God's thoughts for us. It is the discipline of focusing on a verse or verses (in context) for a period of time. Reflecting on specific verses allows our heart to gain practical insight for coping with cancer. Meditation makes possible a healthy mental attitude that in turn affects our body's response to disease.

An important key to Bible meditation is to use the imagination to mentally see each concept in the verse or verses under consideration. When Jesus taught, He frequently used word pictures to communicate spiritual truth. He called Himself the Bread of Life, the Good Shepherd. He told His followers they would be "fishers of men." He spoke of the seed sower and the pearl "of great value."

Nothing was of greater benefit to me in coping with cancer than the choice to daily meditate, to memorize promises in the Scriptures and to pray. When I discovered a helpful Scripture verse, I recorded it on a card. Soon I had a pack of small cards for my meditation during each treatment day.

In order to assist you in realizing the tremendous benefit of this method, I have listed several verses of Scripture under the heading of "Heart-Talk" at the end of each chapter. At the end of the book I have included 12 "Creative Choices" cards with verses. These, too, can be clipped and used for meditation and prayer. You may wish to add verses from the Bible that you personally have discovered.

3. *Realize the Word of God brings life and health*—"[My words] are life . . . and health" (4:22). Here is a great promise to motivate us to faithful meditation and prayer each day. And just as the psalmist prayed that his "meditation be pleasing to [God] as [he] rejoice[d] in the Lord" (Psalm 104:34), so we will experience similar joy in our hearts. Lloyd John Ogilvie in his book, *Making Stress Work for You*, writes:

> Creative meditation includes both prayer for our suffering and praise for the Lord's help in spite of everything. We can talk to him about the difficulties and delights in life. He helps us overcome our hard times of suffering and truly enjoy our times of praise. And soon the praise over His interventions gives us a hopeful resiliency for the future.[2]

4. *Protect your heart with biblical thinking*—"Guard your heart,/ for it is the wellspring of life" (4:23). The emphasis to "guard your heart" is fundamental to life and health. Surrounding our thoughts with the Word of God will increase our faith and form a "shield" with which

we can "extinguish all the flaming arrows" that Satan will hurl against us (Ephesians 6:16).

Thus, our goal is to formulate a pattern of thinking that mirrors biblical teaching. It is essential that we become sensitive to what our heart is saying as we walk daily through the world of cancer. You will find examples of heart-talk and prayer at the end of this and the other chapters. Hopefully they will enable you to work through the heartaches of cancer or gain understanding of the thoughts and feelings of others afflicted with the disease.

Here are five tips to influence your heart-talk through meditation:

1. Set aside a time each day that is as free as possible from distractions.

2. Use that time to memorize and meditate on one verse or passage of Scripture.

3. Consult your Bible concordance and Bible dictionary for further clarity as to what God is saying in the verse or passage.

4. Review the verses you memorized on previous days.

5. Utilize the Word, engrafted in your heart, as you pray.

Use mind, emotions, body to make creative choices

To make creative choices, it is important that

we recognize the priority of the mind within the heart. Notice the biblical order:

First, the mind. "For as he thinks in his heart, so is he" (Proverbs 23:7 NKJ). H. Norman Wright observes the priority of the thought life in relation to the emotions:

> Our thought life is both basic and important. God created us so that our feelings *follow* our thoughts. Many people today, however, have reversed the process and in so doing have a life of instability.[3]

Joan Borysenko, director of Harvard University's Mind/Body Clinic, offers this fact concerning healing through the mind-emotions-body connection:

> Scientists are finding that the areas of the brain that control emotions are also rich in chemical messengers called neuropeptides, which are secreted by the brain, the immune system and other organs.[4]

Our Creator God, through His grace and goodness to all of us, has built into our bodies a means of relieving pain through the interaction of mind and emotions. Positive thoughts not only create positive emotions but they also release a chemical to ease physical pain.

Second, the emotions. "You will keep in perfect peace/ him whose mind is steadfast,/ because he trusts in you" (Isaiah 26:3). Note that the emotion of peace is conditioned upon the mind that chooses to trust in God. *Newsweek* reported this interesting study of the "joy factor":

> One study at the Pittsburgh Cancer Institute . . . found that a factor called "joy"—meaning mental resilience and vigor—was the second strongest predictor of survival time for a group of patients with recurrent breast cancer.[5]

That study is another demonstration of God's common grace and goodness to everyone. People who have healthy mental attitudes that reflect positive emotions have a far greater potential for surviving cancer.

Christian psychologists have discovered a basic truth that is of tremendous help in understanding the place of emotions in relationship to our thoughts:

> The first thing to learn about analyzing our emotions is that we cannot control them directly. The reason is that they are side effects of something else that we can directly command, namely our thoughts.[6]

Third, the will. "Whoever is of a willing heart, let him bring [his gift] as an offering to the Lord" (Exodus 35:5 NKJ). Just as the Israelites could choose to participate in the building of the tabernacle by giving an offering for its construction, so the Lord lets us choose to participate in becoming whole persons. God created us with the freedom to determine how we will respond to the crisis of cancer. Even the paralyzed man in Jesus' day had to make a choice when Jesus asked him, "Do you want to get well?" (John 5:6). He had to choose whether to allow Jesus to heal him or to remain an invalid.

As we consider the will in this process of healing, can we "heart-talk" briefly? Suppose one of my loved ones is faced with cancer, which unsettles my emotions. I feel all loss of control over the situation and cannot foresee the consequences of this cancer. But rather than to permit these emotions to control me, I choose to think biblically on what God says through Isaiah: "You will keep in perfect peace/ him whose mind is steadfast,/ because he trusts in you" (Isaiah 26:3). Thus through the power of choice, I choose the very peace that God offers to me, and I discover that "God himself, the God of peace," begins to "sanctify [me] through and through," keeping "blameless" my "whole spirit, soul and body" (1 Thessalonians 5:23). When I choose to think biblically, my emotions will settle down to experience peace.

Letting go of our negative emotions

Jerry Bridges, vice-president for corporate affairs of The Navigators and author of *Trusting God*, told in *Discipleship* magazine of doctors discovering a large malignant tumor in his wife's abdomen. After eight weeks of radiation therapy, Mrs. Bridges underwent a CAT scan to determine the status of the tumor. The day before she was to learn the results, Mrs. Bridges found herself anxious about the news she would get. How did she cope with her emotions? For some days during that difficult time she had been turning to Psalm 42:11 for assurance:

> Why are you downcast, O my soul?
>   Why so disturbed within me?
> Put your hope in God,
>   for I will yet praise him,
>   my Savior and my God.

Mrs. Bridges said to God, "Lord, I choose not to be downcast; I choose not to be disturbed. I choose to put my trust in You." She related how her feelings did not change immediately, but after a while her heart became calm as she deliberately chose to trust in God.[7]

Heart-Talk

Emotionally (I feel): I feel discouraged and frightened because cancer is too big for me to handle. I am out of control. I feel the sentence of death has been pronounced upon me.

Intellectually (I think): However, I am now filling my thinking with and meditating on the healing Word of God that declares:

> Have I not commanded you? Be strong and courageous. Do not be terrified; do not be discouraged, for the Lord your God will be with you wherever you go. (Joshua 1:9)

> God did not give us a spirit of timidity, but a spirit of power, of love and of self-discipline. (2 Timothy 1:7)

> Who shall separate us from the love of Christ? Shall trouble or hardship or persecution or famine or nakedness or danger or sword? As it is written:
>   "For your sake we face death all day
>   long;
>   we are considered as sheep to be
>   slaughtered."
> No, in all these things we are more than conquerors through him who loved us.
>   (Romans 8:35–37)

Volitionally (I choose): Though I did not choose cancer, I choose to creatively cope with cancer. For I know that God commands me to be strong and courageous. He promises that I can be even more than a conqueror through Him who loves me. I choose this promise to give me the courage to face the world of cancer.

Prayer

Dear Lord, I thank You for the power of choice that You have given me. I desire to use this power to cope courageously with cancer each day. I choose to guard my heart by meditating on Your Word. I pray that Your peace and love will settle my emotions. I believe that through You I can be more than a conqueror during this crisis. In Jesus' name, amen.

"Cancer is a divine appointment to receive Christ's miracle of His life into one's heart."

And this is the testimony: God has given us eternal life, and this life is in his Son. He who has the Son has life; he who does not have the Son of God does not have life.
1 John 5:11–12

Deity indwelling men! That, I say, is Christianity and no man has experienced rightly the power of Christian belief until he has known this for himself as a living reality.[1]
A.W. Tozer

One day as I shared my faith with a housewife, I quoted a familiar verse of Scripture: "All have sinned and fall short of the glory of God" (Romans 3:23). I commented on the verse by saying, "Since the fall of Adam and Eve in the Garden of Eden, all of us, including you and me, are sinners by birth."

The woman looked puzzled. "How," she

asked, "is sin passed down to all of us? Is it through the chromosomes and genes?"

Many people, like that housewife, do not understand that we not only possess a physical body but also a human spirit that has been contaminated by sin. Just as genes pass down their traits from generation to generation, so sin has passed down its traits through the whole human race from generation to generation. Since Adam was humanity's representative, the whole race born to Adam and Eve became plagued with the disease of sin. Sin is an unhealthy condition of the human spirit that affects our whole person.

Our heart needs God

God created Adam with an amazing body. He also designed Adam with the spiritual capacity to allow his heart to be God's dwelling place. In his best-known line from *Confessions,* Augustine wrote, "Thou hast made us for Thyself and our hearts are restless till they find their rest in Thee." It is impossible to experience wholeness and fulfillment in life until we rest in Him.

When Adam, in Eden, rebelled against his Creator, his relationship with God was ended. Adam and Eve's spiritual immune system broke down. The cancer of sin entered their hearts, resulting in spiritual death. When this happened, true love for God gave way to the malignancy of lust, greed and countless forms of selfishness. Adam and Eve themselves seized the empty throne of their inner human hearts, created for God. Instead of directing their worship toward the Creator, they turned inward to themselves, the created. Adam and Eve turned from a God-centered lifestyle and chose to follow one that was self-centered. Their hearts also became infected with the temptations of Satan.

Four characteristics of sin

Sin has four universal characteristics:

1. *Sin is no respecter of persons.* It has infected the whole human family:

> What shall we conclude then? Are we any better? Not at all! We have already made the charge that Jews and Gentiles alike are all under sin. (Romans 3:9)

2. *Sin is uncontrollable without a remedy.* Sin comes in many forms, all of them ugly. Left unchecked, sin goes berserk and wreaks havoc in broken lives and heartache. The Bible lists some of the forms sin takes:

> The acts of the sinful nature are obvious: sexual immortality, impurity and debauchery; idolatry and witchcraft; hatred, discord, jealousy, fits of rage, selfish ambition, dissensions, factions and envy; drunkenness, orgies, and the like. I warn

you, as I did before, that those who live like this will not inherit the kingdom of God. (Galatians 5:19–21)

3. *Sin grips its prey tenaciously.* It makes slaves of people and holds them with an unrelenting grip:

> Don't you know that when you offer yourselves to someone to obey him as slaves, you are slaves to the one whom you obey—whether you are slaves to sin, which leads to death, or to obedience, which leads to righteousness? (Romans 6:16)

4. *Sin, if unchecked, results in death.* The Bible makes it very clear:

> The wages of sin is death, but the gift of God is eternal life in Christ Jesus our Lord. (Romans 6:23)

The sooner we receive help, the sooner we can ward off the reality of impending death. We need a Savior who specializes in providing the only known deliverance from our spiritual death. That Specialist is Jesus Christ, who heals us from the malignancy of sin and offers us eternal life. Jesus Christ is our connection to God for spiritual health and wholeness.

The ABCs of healing from the cancer of sin

A. *Accept the Bible's diagnosis.* Jesus put His finger on your problem when He said:

> From within, out of men's hearts, come evil thoughts, sexual immorality, theft, murder, adultery, greed, malice, deceit, lewdness, envy, slander, arrogance and folly. (Mark 7:21–22)

Without outside assistance, you are in sin's death grip. Sin is uncontrollable. It is terminal.

B. *Believe that Jesus alone can cure you from sin.* Once you are convinced of the reality of Step A, you must move quickly to Step B and decide on the prescribed treatment. The Scriptures are very clear that only Jesus Christ can cure you:

> Salvation is found in no one else, for there is no other name under heaven given to men by which we must be saved. (Acts 4:12)

C. *Confess your sinful state and by faith receive the incredible spiritual healing offered by Jesus Christ.* To confess is "to agree with." Agree with the diagnosis of the Bible that you are helpless to heal yourself of your sinful state. Agree that you can be healed by Jesus, who is able to do for you in a miraculous way what you are un-able to do for yourself. Recognize that you are spiritually dead through Adam and that your human spirit has been controlled by self. Believe that God through Jesus Christ heals your human spirit of the cancer of sin.

This prepares your heart for the Spirit of Christ to come to indwell it. Paul prayed that the believers in Ephesus would know the power that the Christ-centered life brings to face all of life's problems:

> I pray that out of his glorious riches he may strengthen you with power through his Spirit in your inner being, so that Christ may dwell in your hearts through faith. (Ephesians 3:16–17a)

Look at the diagram on the following page. At the top is the self-centered, sinful life passed on by Adam and Eve to all of us, resulting in spiritual death. At the bottom is the Christ-centered, victorious life made possible as we put our faith in Jesus and His death for us on the cross, resulting in eternal life. Surely you wish to be rid of sin, related to Christ and responsive to His will in your life.

Only God Himself through Jesus Christ can heal your sinful human heart and restore the healthful relationship that sin poisoned.

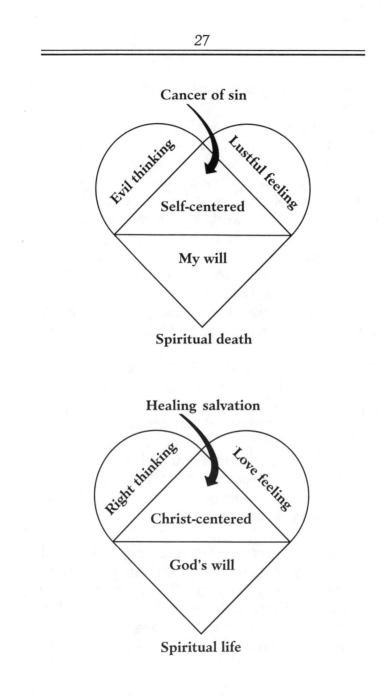

Four striking similarities between cancer and sin

There are four amazing similarities between sin, which we have just looked at, and cancer.

1. *Cancer, like sin, is no respecter of persons.* Cancer can strike young and old, rich and poor, football players and accountants. People in all parts of the world have some form of cancer. It is estimated that a record one million Americans were diagnosed with cancer in 1989. Over the years, cancer will strike three out of four families.

2. *Cancer, like sin, is uncontrollable without a remedy.* The United Cancer Council states:

> A body is made up of billions of normal cells, all of which multiply and divide in an orderly manner to perform their own particular function. Whenever these cells, for some unknown reason, go berserk and grow in a disorderly and chaotic manner, crowding out normal cells and robbing them of nourishment, the condition is known as cancer.[2]

Some cancers are fast growing and spread rapidly in several weeks. Others grow more slowly over several years. There are over 200 forms of cancer. Left unchecked, cancer takes over the human body, wreaking physical and psychological havoc.

3. *Cancer, like sin, grips its prey with tenacity.*
Hippocrates first identified cancer about 400
B.C. He coined the term *karkinoma,* meaning
"crab" for the malignant tumors. The Latin
word for *crab, cancrum,* was later the basis for
our word *cancer.* Cancer, like a crab, grabs hold
of its prey with a tremendous tenacity, just as
sin does.

4. *Cancer, like sin, if left unchecked, brings
death.* The American Cancer Society puts it
very bluntly:

> Cancer is a group of diseases in which
> there is uncontrolled growth of abnormal
> cells, which if unchecked will cause death.

Along with the 1,040,000 new cancer cases
for 1990, the American Cancer Society
projected 510,000 cancer deaths. The projec-
tions included 142,000 deaths from new lung
cancer, 60,900 deaths from colon-rectal cancer,
44,000 deaths from female breast cancer and
30,000 deaths from prostate cancer.[3]
The sooner a cancerous condition receives
treatment, the better the patient's chances of
recovery.

Other similarities between cancer and sin

There are still other similarities between cancer, which attacks the physical body, and sin,
which attacks the spirit.

In both cases, the victim is in great distress be-

cause of a condition he or she is personally helpless to cure. Outside help is needed to save the person.

In both cases, another person must act on behalf of the sufferer to deliver him or her. For the cancer victim, it is the oncologist, hospital personnel and others involved in the healing process. For the sinner, it is Jesus Christ, the God-man who enfleshed Himself and lived among us a life without sin. In this unique position He had the infinite power of God to act on behalf of the sufferers. Thus He was able to deliver from sin and impart spiritual life.

The action of the deliverer brings release. Frequently the best efforts of medicine fail to deliver the cancer sufferer. But Jesus' deliverance through His death on the cross is 100 percent effective for all who call upon Him in faith. He releases us from our unhealthy sinful state and gives new life and power so that we can be righteous. Peter declares:

> He himself bore our sins in his body on the tree, so that we might die to sins and live for righteousness; by his wounds you have been healed. (1 Peter 2:24)

Five responses to the diagnosis

Whether sin or cancer, when we are given the diagnosis, and a certain program of treatment is recommended, we can respond in five ways:

1. *Denial.* Many people deny they have cancer. "There must be some mistake," they say. "Perhaps the lab made an error and got the names mixed up." Some pretend that cancer does not exist in them.

When presented with the Bible's diagnosis that everyone has the cancer of sin, many people will deny it also. Most of this group are led to believe in the inherent goodness of human nature. Large numbers are so engrossed in materialism that they are indifferent to their spiritual state.

2. *Despair.* Others react with an attitude of hopelessness. "There is no use," they say. "I'm too far gone." Unfortunately, those who give up pay the consequences.

In the spiritual realm, people react similarly. "I'm too great a sinner." "My past life has been too wicked." It is difficult for these to realize that Christ is able to give them eternal life and spiritual healing however dark their past has been.

3. *Procrastination.* "I'll wait a while and see what happens." "Let me think about it first." They may be too busy with goals yet unfulfilled to want to stop for treatment. This reaction also is typical of those who are confronted with the diagnosis of sin. Alas, this tragic mind-set results in permanent spiritual death.

4. *Seek alternatives.* "I saw a magazine ad for a new treatment." "A friend told me about this doctor in Greece . . . ." Such a decision leads to

quackery. Many promise quick fixes and miraculous recoveries. They leave in their dust a host of deceived and heartbroken victims.

When it comes to sin, there is no lack of cults certifying that their brand of treatment is the only way to heaven. Even the occult, sometimes in the guise of psychology, is hard-selling its cures for our spiritual ills. The Bible warns:

> Dear friends, do not believe every spirit, but test the spirits to see whether they are from God, because many false prophets have gone out into the world. This is how you can recognize the Spirit of God: Every spirit that acknowledges that Jesus Christ has come in the flesh is from God, but every spirit that does not acknowledge Jesus is not from God. (1 John 4:1–3a)

5. *Submit to the experts.* I came to a decision to receive chemotherapy. It was prescribed by the staff of experienced medical doctors who employed all of the available technology to arrive at their conclusion.

The Bible—the Word of God—gives us the only correct solution to heal us of the malignant cancer of sin:

> If you will confess with your mouth, "Jesus is Lord," and believe in your heart that God raised him from the dead, you will be saved. For it is with your heart that you

believe and are justified, and it is with your mouth that you confess and are saved. (Romans 10:9–10)

"Please sign the consent form"

I accepted the diagnosis of the oncologists. I was in great distress and unable to help myself. I signed the consent form necessary for the doctors to begin treatment. From there on, the doctors acted on my behalf. They did for me what I could not do for myself.

If you have not received Christ Jesus into your life, accept without further delay His offer to heal you of the cancer of sin. Do not deny your sin. Do not feel you are hopeless. Do not put off the treatment. Do not try some other method. Agree with the diagnosis and submit yourself to Jesus, the Great Physician.

If you want to make this life-changing decision, meditate on the Heart-Talk that follows and offer the prayer you will find there. Then sign your name and include the date on the consent form at the end of this chapter.

Heart-Talk

Emotionally (I feel): I feel shaken and insecure because I am unsure of my future. I feel helpless to save myself from sin. My emotions are working overtime. I am anxious to examine my relationship with God.

Intellectually (I think): I am now filling my thinking with the healing Word of God that declares five important truths necessary for salvation:

1. *Jesus' work on the cross alone can save me from sin.*

> What I received I passed on to you as of first importance: that Christ died for our sins according to the Scriptures, that he was buried, that he was raised on the third day. (1 Corinthians 15:3–4)

2. *Repentance of sin and faith in Jesus alone save me.*

> I have declared to both Jews and Greeks that they must turn to God in repentance and have faith in our Lord Jesus. (Acts 20:21)

3. *God's gift of salvation is offered to me by grace and not by works.*

> It is by grace you have been saved, through faith—and this not from yourselves, it is a gift of God—not by works, so that no one can boast. (Ephesians 2:8–9)

4. *Eternal life is given to me when I receive God's Son.*

This is the testimony: God has given us eternal life, and this life is in his Son. He who has the Son has life; he who does not have the Son of God does not have life. (1 John 5:11–12)

5. *It is God's desire that Christ should dwell in my heart.*

I pray that out of his glorious riches he may strengthen you with power through his Spirit in your inner being, so that Christ may dwell in your hearts through faith. (Ephesians 3:16–17a)

Volitionally (I choose): I believe with my whole heart God's plan of salvation as given above. Thus, I will repeat the prayer below. I will repent of my sins and receive Jesus into my heart.

Prayer
Dear Lord Jesus, I thank You for dying on the cross to save me from my sins. I have led a self-centered life, but I am determined to live a Christ-centered life. I repent of my sins and my self-centered life. I now receive You into my heart. I am grateful that my heart is now the dwelling place of God. In Jesus' name, amen.

CONSENT FORM

To permit Jesus, the Great Physician, to:

1. cleanse and heal my heart from all sin.
2. dwell within my heart as my Savior and Lord.
3. grant me the wonderful gift of spiritual life.

Name_____Date_____

I have God's assurance that I have spiritual life according to God's Word. I have Jesus in my heart and have become the dwelling place of God. Now I have the inner power of God to cope with cancer.

This is the testimony: God has given us eternal life, and this life is in his Son. He who has the Son has life; he who does not have the Son of God does not have life.

I write these things to you who believe in the name of the Son of God so that you may know that you have eternal life. (1 John 5:11–13)

"Since our sovereign Lord permits cancer for His glory and our spiritual growth, I will glorify God and grow."

"For I know the plans I have for you,"
declares the Lord, "plans to prosper you and
not to harm you, plans to give you hope and
a future." Jeremiah 29:11

A true recognition of God's sovereignty
causes us to hold our plans in abeyance to
God's will. It makes us recognize that the
Divine Potter has absolute power over the
clay and molds it according to his own im-
perial pleasure.[1] A.W. Pink

Following the church service in which the diagnosis of my advanced cancer was announced, one of the men confronted me.

"Pastor," he said, "I'm mad at God. Why did God let you get cancer? You are such a good person. You don't deserve to have cancer. Why didn't a bad person get it instead of you?"

Four years later, in a restaurant, I shared my testimony of healing with a former neighbor whom I had not seen in years. She asked, "Why did God allow you to be healed of cancer and not a pastor whom many of our churches prayed for faithfully? We believed he would be healed, but he died."

How does a person answer the difficult "why" questions? To be creative, we must dispense with the "why" questions and substitute some "what" questions. *What does God want me to learn from this that will result in my spiritual growth? What may I do through this to glorify God?* Questions like those are helpful as we recognize that God has allowed cancer for our spiritual growth and His glory. If you are a cancer patient or one who is trying to encourage someone who is, remember those two creative "what" questions. The "why" question asked by the angry church member did not encourage me to grow and glorify God. And the answer to the "why" question of my former neighbor regarding life and death is known only to God.

When tested by adversity, I find myself often praying, "Lord, here I am again. What are you trying to teach me this time? May I learn the lesson well the first time!"

The Lord is Lord of all or not Lord at all

On this side of eternity we cannot fully understand the answers to the "why" questions. The best understanding possible with our

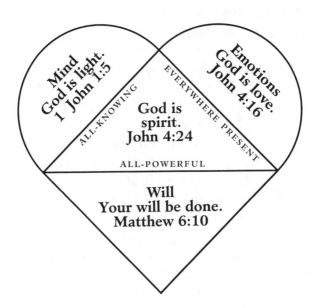

human limitations is embodied in the doctrine of the sovereignty of God (see diagram above). The term expresses the supreme rulership of God. He planned, created and sustains this vast universe by His divine will. He possesses all power and no one can defeat His counsels nor can anyone frustrate His purposes. Ancient Job, who had more reason than most of us for supposing that life was treating him unfairly, instead said of God's supreme power:

> I know that you can do all things;
>   No plan of yours can be thwarted.
>   (Job 42:2)

The prophet Isaiah delivered this message of God's sovereign power for Israel to fix in its national mind and heart:

> Remember the former things, those of
>   long ago;
>   I am God, and there is no other;
>   I am God, and there is none like me.
> I make known the end from the beginning,
>   from ancient times, what is still to come.
> I say: My purpose will stand,
>   and I will do all that I please.
>   (Isaiah 46:9–10)

The bottom line, which cancer patients and their families ought to take to heart, is that the sovereign, all-powerful God of the universe has the right to plan and do all that He pleases to do. W.C. Doughty shares this insight:

> It is not a negation of faith to recognize the sovereignty of God's will in relation to your sicknesses and healing; rather it is an acknowledgement that as your Lord, he has a right to deal with you in your body as he wills.[2]

The goodness of God
What is reassuring about God's sovereignty is that God always works in accord with His character. One of His character traits is goodness.

He is a good God. Holiness, justice, mercy, love, grace and truth are elements of His goodness. When we realize that all of His plans, decisions and judgments are the outcome of these qualities, should it be easy to be angry with Him or difficult to submit to Him?

Furthermore, God takes us through crises in order for us to develop a closer personal relationship with Him as our heavenly Father. In terms of personal relationships, the ultimate description of God is Father. It is our heavenly Father's pleasure that we recognize that He deals with us according to all the facets of His divine goodness.

As believers, we should find it comforting to know that God is at work behind every adverse circumstance for our spiritual growth. It pleases the Father when we use our freedom in Christ to grow in love, grace, holiness, justice, mercy and truth. In expressing this freedom to grow, Larry O. Richards shares this insight:

> We have been shaped by God to love Him and to enjoy Him forever. Only by choosing to serve God can we become the people we were created to be. This freedom to experience our destiny is a wonderful freedom indeed. Only when you and I willingly submit to the lordship of Jesus Christ can we learn what freedom truly is.[3]

Sovereignty, sickness, Satan and the Savior

Sickness entered the world ultimately as a result of mankind's sin. We see in the Bible, however, that individual diseases may have various causes. I want to briefly examine several of these with you.

In the book of Exodus, we see diseases as a divine judgment inflicted upon the Egyptians of that era. God said:

> If you listen carefully to the voice of the Lord your God and do what is right in his eyes, if you pay attention to his commandments and keep all his decrees, I will not bring on you any of the diseases I brought on the Egyptians, for I am the Lord, who heals you. (Exodus 15:26)

From that admonition and promise, we can learn three important truths:

1. God, not Satan, brought disease upon the Egyptians of that era.

2. God promised immunity to the diseases He inflicted upon the Egyptians if Israel would "pay attention to his commandments and keep all his decrees."

3. God reveals His nature as both Healer and Protector. As Protector He said, "I will not bring on you any of the diseases I brought on the Egyptians." As Healer He said, "I am the

Lord, who heals you." Later Israel would sing about these benefits:

> Praise the Lord, O my soul,
>   and forget not all his benefits—
> who forgives all your sins
>   and heals all your diseases,
> who redeems your life from the pit
>   and crowns you with love and
> compassion. (Psalm 103:2–4)

Disease can also be inflicted by Satan, as seen in the familiar story of Job, alluded to above. God in His sovereignty permitted Satan to take away Job's wealth, to destroy his children and to afflict Job with intensely painful boils. But there was purpose in what God permitted. Job was proud of his righteousness and defensive of his status. After God finished dealing with Job (chapters 38–41), the patriarch capitulated.

> My ears had heard of you,
>   but now my eyes have seen you.
> Therefore I despise myself
>   and repent in dust and ashes. (42:5–6)

God concluded the test by rewarding Job with double of everything he had had previously. Affliction resulted in Job's spiritual growth and in God receiving glory.

In the New Testament there are two examples of Satan afflicting persons. Luke recounts the healing by Jesus of a woman severely "bent over" and unable to stand erect, "whom Satan [had] kept bound for eighteen long years" (Luke 13:16). The apostle Paul had "a thorn in [his] flesh, a messenger of Satan, to torment [him]" (2 Corinthians 12:7). Although he does not further identify the "thorn," it quite certainly was a physical affliction.

In some instances of diseases mentioned in the Bible, neither God nor Satan are mentioned as being behind the affliction—for example, the stroke that felled the Shunammite couple's son (2 Kings 4:18–21) or Naaman's leprosy (2 Kings 5:1). In the case of the man blind from birth (John 9:1), disease was inflicted to bring glory to God. Jesus corrected His disciples when they supposed the man's blindness had to be blamed either on the sins of his parents or on his own sins. " 'Neither this man nor his parents sinned,' said Jesus, 'but this happened so that the work of God might be displayed in his life' " (John 9:3).

God in His divine plan sent Jesus to this sin-cursed earth "to destroy the devil's work" (1 John 3:8). For that reason Jesus died. For that reason He rose from the dead. For that reason He will return to complete the work He was sent to accomplish.

Just like a lump of clay

Job had to learn the lesson of unquestioning

submission the hard way. And Job's descendants are cut from the same cloth. Paul asks:

> Who are you, O man, to talk back to God? "Shall what is formed say to him who formed it, 'Why did you make me like this?'" [quoting from Isaiah 29:16 and 45:9]. Does not the potter have the right to make out of the same lump of clay some pottery for noble purposes and some for common use? (Romans 9:20–21)

A deaconess in one of my former churches told me she had a lump of clay on her bedroom dresser. When she went to bed at night and when she arose in the morning, it reminded her that she was just like a lump of clay in the Potter's hands. She recognized God's absolute power over her daily life. She humbly submitted her life to the divine Potter to mold it according to His goodness.

My personal onset of cancer

I must confess that I experienced a brief spiritual tailspin when the diagnosis of cancer was first given to me. It was the "Why me?" question, and I found it a difficult pill to swallow—that God should permit me to contract cancer. But my stunned heart became more pliable as my mind began to center on the sovereignty of God. I determined to allow the divine Potter to use this unwanted cancer for

His glory and my growth. I needed to learn submission to His molding hand in all of the unpleasant daily details associated with the tests and treatments.

May I share with you briefly my experiences leading up to and immediately following the cancer diagnosis? In December, 1980, I developed a bronchial condition, which doctors treated during the following three months. Medications included three courses of antibiotics, including penicillin and ampicillin, which did not resolve the problem. But I did shed 20 unneeded pounds!

At night I began to experience chills followed by profuse perspiration. Two or three times during the night my bed sheets and pajamas had to be changed. I had a fever of 102 degrees. On March 4, my 49th birthday, I made my fourth and last visit to the local doctor. By that time my energy level had decreased to the point where I gasped for air when walking up a few stairs. The coughing continued.

On March 11, my wife Elaine and I drove to the University of Michigan Hospital, 21 miles from Wayne, our home at the time. X-rays showed an abnormal lung condition. Doctors, suspecting tuberculosis, admitted me to the Medicine Pulmonary Clinic, placing me in isolation. They gave me oxygen to assist me in breathing.

It was a situation to test and refine my faith. Instead of standing next to hospital beds, encouraging the faith of others, as I had done for so many years as a pastor, I now found myself the patient. I was determined to glorify God by being a good patient. In my ministry I had been inspired by Christians who rose above physical disability with a joyful attitude. I had visited them to bring encouragement and went away encouraged myself by their faith in God. They were now my role models. Would I follow their example and glorify God? Would I, too, experience the spiritual growth they had experienced? A series of medical tests soon would answer that question.

Faith tested during the hospital tests

The thoracentesis was a procedure performed in my hospital room. I was instructed to sit up on the side of the bed. The doctor stood on the other side, behind me, a needle two to three inches in length in hand. After administering a local anaesthetic to the lower section of my back to deaden the pain, he inserted the needle into the pleura sac that encases the lungs. The purpose, the doctor said, was two-fold. During the course of an infectious disease, the pleura sac fills with fluid, compressing the lungs. Draining off the fluid relieves the pressure, easing breathing. Also, the fluid can be analyzed to determine a more accurate diagnosis of the disease. The doctor informed me that the danger of the procedure, although remote, was to penetrate too deeply, puncturing the lung.

Alarm! This was a call to pray! In my heart I prayed earnestly that the Great Physician would guide the doctor's hand throughout the entire procedure. And God answered with His peace. I felt His presence and knew that He was behind the scene controlling the doctor's hand. The procedure was completed without mishap, for which I praised the Lord. By the grace of God I had endured the first test.

Responding to the cancer bombshell

The most difficult test came when we got the results. My wife and I waited anxiously through most of the next day. Finally, late in the afternoon, two sober-faced doctors entered the room.

"We are very sorry to have to give you this report," one of them began apologetically. "The fluid taken from your pleura sac showed cancer cells."

The word *cancer* struck terror within me. Momentarily I was overwhelmed with disbelief. As my imagination worked overtime, I struggled to keep my composure. Fear of surgery, pain, tubes, disability and death swept over me. I wanted to escape. I wanted to think all of this was just a bad dream. I could identify with the psalmist who cried out:

My heart is in anguish within me;

the terrors of death assail me.
Fear and trembling have beset me;
  horror has overwhelmed me.
I said, "Oh, that I had the wings of a dove!
  I would fly away and be at rest—
I would flee far away." (Psalm 55:4–7a)

During my brief bout of inner turmoil the two doctors were doing their best to assure us that the university had the experience and resources to give the best treatment possible. Although the tests were not conclusive, the doctors suspected lymphoma. Certain forms of lymphoma were treatable, and treatments had resulted in remission.

Elaine stayed with me the rest of the evening. She was very supportive, doing her best to encourage me. I was concerned for her welfare and that of our sons. We did not own a home. On my modest salary I had had no opportunity to make financial provision for their future.

Then the ultimate "why" question hit me. Less than a year before that, by dint of prolonged, intensive effort, I had completed doctoral studies. Why had the Lord permitted me to spend all that time and energy on a doctorate only to cut me down at the prime age of 49? Elaine urged me to be positive and to exercise faith in the Word of God. Six months earlier, I had claimed for my mid-life a verse from the book of Job: "The Lord blessed the latter part of Job's life more than the first (42:12a).

The context informs us that God had blessed
Job with twice what he had had before his affliction. Now Elaine and I agreed together in
prayer that we would battle the cancer and
believe God for a double portion of blessed
ministry in this latter part of life.

The American hostages had recently been
released by Iran, and Elaine remind me of
Katherine Koob, who was held for 444 days. In
her confinement Miss Koob had the confidence that one day she would go free. She
based her hope on verses from Psalm 118:

> "I will not die but live,
>   and will proclaim what the Lord has
>   done.
> The Lord has chastened me severely,
>   but he has not given me over to death.
>   (verses 17–18)

Elaine and I agreed that I must not allow
myself to be a hostage to the negative thoughts
that lead to depression and hopelessness. I
would exercise positive faith in the promises of
God for healing and ministry. The Lord loved
me. The proof of His love was His discipline,
"because the Lord disciplines those he loves"
(Hebrews 12:6). This discipline was for my personal development in Christlikeness. Through
it I desired to learn the lessons I needed to
know. God had not given me over to death, but
I would live and declare His works. Elaine and

I would be blessed with a greater ministry than we had experienced the first half of our lives.

Like fall leaves on a windy day, the negative, destructive thoughts of the old nature blew away. They were replaced by the positive, constructive promises in the Word of God. We determined, by the grace of God, to go forward in positive faith, toward recovery.

Severe shaping on the Potter's wheel

In order to win the war, battles must be fought. As battles progress, they tend to become more intense. Victory is at the price of resolve and faith.

The next day I was scheduled for an examination of my ears and throat. The young student doctor had no problem until he tried to insert down my throat a small mirror on a long handle. He instructed me to stick out my tongue, which he wrapped with gauze and held while he tried unsuccessfully six times to look into my throat. Each time I gagged. Finally he gave up and called for help. The more experienced doctor instructed me to take short exhaling and inhaling breaths.

"When you are on the verge of gagging," he said, "give a high-pitched 'E-e-e-e-e-e.' " I gladly cooperated with the highest "E-e-e-e-e-e" I could muster. It was not loud, but it worked. After a few squeaky sounds, the test was over.

"Your left vocal cord is paralyzed," the doctor said, putting the mirror to one side as he faced me eye-to-eye. "The nerve that loops down from the vocal chord seems to have pressure on it. That compressed nerve is paralyzing your left vocal chord."

How can I preach with partially paralyzed vocal cords? How can a preacher communicate if he doesn't have a voice? Immediately, the negative lights began flashing. But rather than dwell on the negative, I looked at Isaiah 43:18–19 and jotted these verses on a 3" by 5" card:

> Forget the former things;
>   do not dwell on the past.
> See, I am doing a new thing!
>   Now it springs up; do you not perceive
>   it?
> I am making a way in the desert
>   and streams in the wasteland.

Heart-Talk

Emotionally (I feel): I feel angry with God, for I don't understand why I have been diagnosed with cancer. I just can't believe that it is true. I feel hurt that God has allowed me to contract cancer and am frustrated that my plans are interrupted. I fear suffering, and I am worried about dying.

Intellectually (I think): I am filling my thoughts with and meditating on the healing Word of God that tells me:

"I know the plans I have for you," declares the Lord, "plans to prosper you and not to harm you, plans to give you hope and a future." (Jeremiah 29:11)

The eternal God is your refuge,
   and underneath are the everlasting arms.
(Deuteronomy 33:27a)

Do not worry about tomorrow, for tomorrow will worry about itself. Each day has enough trouble of its own. (Matthew 6:34)

Be strong in the Lord and in his mighty power. (Ephesians 6:10)

Whether you eat or drink or whatever you do, do it all for the glory of God. (1 Corinthians 10:31)

Volitionally (I choose): I choose to view this crisis in the light of the sovereignty of God. I refuse to waste my time on the "why" question. Instead, I shall ask God, "What are You going to teach me?" I believe the Lord is able to heal me according to His divine sovereign will. I choose to grow in love, holiness, justice, mercy, grace and truth and will glorify God in this crisis.

Prayer
I worship You, Heavenly Father, as the

sovereign Lord of the universe. I am a lump of clay in Your hands. Mold me according to Your will. I am ready to learn the lessons You want me to learn so I may grow and bring glory to You. I commit the healing of my whole person completely to You. In Jesus' name I pray, amen.

"Because Christ's death on the wondrous cross is the basis for divine healing, I choose His supernatural power to supplement my doctor's treatments."

He himself bore our sins in his body on the tree, so that we might die to sins and live for righteousness; by his wounds you have been healed. 1 Peter 2:24

When I survey the wondrous cross
On which the Prince of glory died,
My richest gain I count but loss,
And pour contempt on all my pride.
Isaac Watts

The Christian who embraces the healing benefits of the cross for body, soul and spirit has a great advantage over the nonbeliever. The nonbeliever has medical science, psychology and his or her own inner willpower to cope with cancer. The Christian has all of the above plus the added advantage of the conscious child-Father relationship with God who has made available the healing provisions of the cross. The believer knows that God loves His children and has the assurance that the Heavenly Father will not give stones for bread.

Dr. Robert G. Witty, founder of Luther Rice Seminary and president when I studied there, presented these advantages of the Christian over the unbeliever:

> Think of the multiple benefits. The Christian has received God-given physical and spiritual procedures for healthy living. The Christian experiences the inward assistance of the Holy Spirit. God's indwelling presence enables him to obey God's health-giving, spirit-maturing teachings. God's indwelling presence also sustains him in sickness. The unsaved have only human and material help. The Christian has all of the earthly helps, but over and beyond all these, the believer has the presence, the promises and the provisions of his Heavenly Father.[1]

Let me continue my personal testimony begun in the last chapter. I think it demonstrates the advantages the believer possesses in creatively coping with cancer.

Doctors remove a lymph node

A week had passed since I entered the hospital. I was scheduled to have a lymph node at the base of my neck removed. Hematologists at the hospital agreed that a biopsy of the node would determine my type of cancer.

Attendants took me to the operating room, where I was prepped and draped with a sheet from my neck down. Under a local anaesthetic, the surgeon and his assistant retracted a muscle covering the left external jugular vein. Moving the jugular to one side brought a large lymph node into view. This they removed and sent for cultures. My medical report had this comment: "The patient tolerated the procedure well and was taken to his room without any complications."

The next day the assisting surgeon came to my room to check on me.

"You were a good patient," she said. "You had presence of self."

"It was not the presence of self but the presence of God that strengthened me," I responded. "I prayed for you as you performed the biopsy. I mentally sang hymns and quoted Scripture that helped me keep my thoughts off the surgery." She smiled.

Praying, quoting Scripture promises and singing praises are advantages Christians have beyond medicine. These advantages strengthened me throughout all the testing.

One test that gave me ample opportunity for praying, quoting Scripture and singing was the four-hour lymphangiogram. This procedure begins with a pain-deadening injection between the large and second toe on each foot. Then slits are cut on the top of each foot and a dye is injected in the slits to illuminate the lymphatic system on X-ray. Over and over in my mind I sang:

> Cheer up, ye saints of God, there's
> nothing to worry about,
> Nothing to make you feel afraid, nothing
> to make you doubt,
> Remember, Jesus never fails, so why not
> stand up and shout?
> You'll be sorry you worried at all tomorrow
> morning![2]

After two weeks of intensive tests, one of the doctors came into my room to share the results. It was a tense, anxious moment.

"You have diffuse histiocytic lymphoma in the advanced stage," he said. "We recommend that you undergo a series of chemotherapy treatments, but we cannot guarantee any success for recovery." Talk about feeling the sentence of death, as the apostle Paul expressed it in First Corinthians 1:9!

Less than a month to live

To my wife, the oncologist was even more

pessimistic. He told her my cancer was a fast-acting type of lymphoma. Already the malignancy had spread throughout the lymphatic system. X-rays also showed a possible obstruction of the left kidney. He estimated I had less than a month to live.

One of the great advantages of being a Christian is the prayer support from churches and friends. By this time I had received many letters, cards and telephone calls offering encouragement and assuring me of people's prayers. What do you say to a loved one who has been diagnosed as having cancer? Amy Harwell wrote these seven steps in her book, *When Your Friend Gets Cancer*:[3]

1. Check your attitudes about cancer and about friendship.
2. Reach out immediately and boldly.
3. Get prepped on cancer facts and feeling.
4. Offer your helping hands.
5. Share your healing heart.
6. Help your friend make death and dying decisions (if asked).
7. Be there for your friend.

My district superintendent, the Rev. C. David Mangham, sent a letter to all the churches in our district:

Please pray, and ask your people to pray.

John Packo is just 49 years old. It was only last May that he completed his studies and was awarded the Doctor of Ministries degree from Luther Rice Seminary. It would appear that he is just in the prime of his life and ministry. He could surely have many years of fruitful, abounding ministry if God will rebuke this disease.

The Rev. William F. Bryan, senior pastor of the Toledo (Ohio) Gospel Tabernacle, wrote perceptive words that drove me to my knees to seek the will of God for my life:

> Our gracious Lord has not told us to pray that He might mock us, so let us remember that both His promises and His power are manifested for His glory and our comfort. I'm sure we should be resigned to the will of God (even to death) if we are sure of His will. Until He indicates our sickness is unto death, however, surely He is pleased when we search our hearts and then take His promises literally.

I had never heard prayer referred to in just this manner. Certainly prayer was not enjoined upon us so that God might mock us. God's answers do come through the promises in His Word. And I did desire the will of God. If His will was death at this point, I was ready. But as

I searched my heart, I was reminded of my mid-life verse:

> The Lord blessed the latter part of Job's life more than the first. (Job 42:12a)

The Lord spoke to my conscience through that verse with an arresting question: "Didn't I promise to bless your latter life more than the first?"

I answered back in my prayer, "Yes, Lord, but how can I be blessed in later life? I am dying!"

At that moment it occurred to me: *If the Lord gave me that verse, promising a latter life, as my mid-life verse, I was going to live!* With a renewed faith in the promise of God, I believed He would work in my body with my highest spiritual interest at heart.

Looking back on this cancer experience, I am grateful for the added advantages made possible through the wondrous cross of Christ. The believer is given the provisions and presence of a loving heavenly Father who equips us to cope with crises such as cancer. And if God's will is sickness unto death, the believer has a wonderful advantage over the unbeliever. He or she is going to heaven! What a great advantage! The Christian cannot lose! "To live is Christ and to die is gain" (Philippians 1:21).

Healing is rooted in Old Testament redemption

In order to experience the added advantage of holistic healing that goes beyond medical science, it is helpful to review the development of Old Testament healing that had its culmination in the atoning death of Jesus Christ, the Great Physician.

Our heavenly Father revealed Himself as Jehovah—the redemptive name of God. Note in the left hand column of the diagram below the seven compound names of Jehovah. These reveal God's provision for us in redemption. Notice in the right hand column the complete identification of Jesus with these redemptive provisions:

Jehovah of the Old Testament	*Jesus of the New Testament*
Jehovah-Shamma: "The Lord is there or present" (Ezekiel 48:35).	Jesus said, "I am with you always" (Matthew 28:20).
Jehovah-Shalom: "The Lord our peace" (Judges 6:23–24).	Jesus said, "Peace I leave with you" (John 14:27).
Jehovah-Ra-ah: "The Lord is my Shepherd" (Psalm 23:1).	Jesus said, "I am the good Shepherd" (John 10:11).
Jehovah-Jireh: "The Lord will provide [an offering]" (Genesis 22:14).	Jesus: "So Christ was sacrificed once to bear sin" (Hebrews 9:28).

Jehovah-Nissi: "The Lord is my banner" (Exodus 17:15). (We experience victory under Him.)	Jesus: "He gives us the victory through our Lord Jesus Christ" (1 Corinthians 1:30).
Jehovah-Rapha: "I am the Lord, who heals you" (Exodus 15:26).	Jesus: "And [He] healed all the sick" (Matthew 8:16).

The name *Jehovah-Rapha* indicates that God is a healing God. The context of Exodus 15:26 makes it very clear that God is speaking of healing physical diseases. Physical healing is one of the seven redemptive provisions offered by Jehovah God. Isaiah looked forward to the coming of God in human flesh and said:

> Surely he took up our infirmities . . .
> and by his wounds we are healed.
> (Isaiah 53:4–5)

When Jesus died on the cross, He provided physical as well as spiritual redemption. Most of us accept Jesus as our ever-present Companion, our Peace, our Shepherd, our Sacrifice, our victorious Leader and our Righteousness. Is it not reasonable to accept Him as Jehovah-Rapha, "the Lord who heals"?

Jesus Christ provides physical healing
Two principle passages of Scripture bridge the Old and New Testament teaching about

holistic healing. I have already referred to Isaiah's prophecy:

> Surely he took up our infirmties
>   and carried our sorrows,
> yet we considered him stricken by God,
>   smitten by him, and afflicted.
> But he was pierced for our transgressions,
>   he was crushed for our iniquities;
> the punishment that brought us peace was
>   upon him,
>   and by his wounds we are healed.
>   (Isaiah 53:4–5)

Matthew, the New Testament apostle, wrote of the fulfillment of that Old Testament prophecy:

> When evening came, many who were demon-possessed were brought to him, and he drove out the spirits with a word and healed all the sick. This was to fulfill what was spoken through the prophet Isaiah:
> "He took up our infirmities
>   and carried our diseases."
>   (Matthew 8:16–17)

In the context of those verses in Matthew 8, the evangelist observed Jesus healing a leper (8:2–3), a paralyzed servant (8:5–13), Peter's sick mother-in-law (8:14–15) and two demon-possessed men (8:28–33). In the middle of these examples of Jesus' healing ministry, Matthew quoted from Isaiah's well-known prophecy. Thus, he was moved by the Spirit of God to see the healing ministry of Jesus as a fulfillment of what Isaiah had prophesied.

Clearly, Jesus Christ bore our sicknesses in the very same way He bore our sins. He not only made atonement for our sins, but He removed them by His precious blood shed on the cross. So with our physical sicknesses.

Peter, following Christ's death and resurrection, preached holistic healing through the cross:

> He himself bore our sins in his body on the tree, so that we might die to sins and live for righteousness; by his wounds you have been healed. (1 Peter 2:24)

The Greek word for *healed* used by Peter in the above verse refers to physical healing. Peter saw physical healing as having been provided by Christ's death on the cross.

No guarantee of perfection in this life

All of the redemptive benefits achieved by Jesus on the cross are subject to our present state of imperfection. We have no guarantee of perfect holistic health in this life, but God does assure us of perfection in the life to come at the resurrection.

The fact that some people—even some sincere Christians—fail to find the healing that Jesus died to achieve has caused many to reject the idea of holistic health. The fact is that they misunderstand the nature of divine healing. A.J. Gordon, an outstanding 19th century minister and educator, presented a balanced view of divine healing, summarized by Dr. Keith M. Bailey in his book, *Divine Healing: The Children's Bread:*

> Gordon understood that the benefit, like other redemptive benefits, could be claimed and enjoyed to the extent a redeemed man's present state will permit. The benefit of healing in the atonement does not demand that all who exercise faith must have perfect health any more than the benefit of salvation in the atonement demands that all who believe must manifest complete sinlessness.[4]

A clue to our present state of imperfection is found in Genesis 2:17. It reads literally, "Dying, you shalt die." At the moment Adam sinned, death began to work in him. Physical death could have arrived at any moment, as it can with us. Eventually, declining physical abilities bring old age and physical death. Believers who have experienced a healing in their bodies still have death at work within them, although they may experience a new degree of strength and health. Holistic healing, bought for us by Jesus on the cross, becomes clearer when we see sin, sickness and death in terms of positional, experiential and ultimate processes. In his book, *Understanding Divine Healing*, Richard Sipley, who was my former pastor, has a helpful chart (see next page).[5]

Four sources of disease in an imperfect world

Using the term *disease* in its generic sense as any performance-impairing condition of the physical body, there are four major causes:

1. *So-called accidents.* We can fall and break a leg, stumble and tear a ligament, crash in an auto and bruise our body.

2. *Our minds and emotions.* We can make ourselves physically sick through such psychological stresses as anger, worry, depression, bitterness. Doctors acknowledge that much of their practice involves people whose illnesses are directly or indirectly related to stress.

3. *Infections.* Viruses and other microorganisms, penetrating the body's defenses, find an environment where they can multiply, impairing the function of vital parts or systems. Frequently these alien microbes gain access because people break the natural laws of health, eating improperly, not observing essential sanitation, getting insufficient rest.

4. *Supernatural.* God may impose disease because of disobedience (Deuteronomy 28); op-

Through Christ Jesus
the law of the Spirit of life
set me free
from the law of sin and death.
Romans 8:2

The Problem	**SIN**: Both the principle and actions.	**DEATH**: Both the principle and sickness.
Positionally	Sin is forgiven and destroyed. We are declared righteous by the imputed righteousness of Christ.	Death is both removed and destroyed. We are declared deathless by the impartation of eternal life in Christ.
Experientially	We still have sin in us. We still commit sins. We may have forgiveness and victory over sin and sins.	We still have dying bodies. We still get sick. We may have strength and/or healing and victory over our dying bodies.
Completely	At the return of Christ, we will be made like Christ, perfect in holiness for all eternity.	At the return of Christ, we will be made like Christ, being given glorified, perfect bodies for all eternity.

position to His truth (e.g. Elymas the sorcerer, Acts 13:8); sinful behavior (e.g. the Corinthian church members, 1 Corinthians 11:30); or to discipline us to produce "a harvest of righteousness" (Hebrews 12:11) or "so that the work of God might be displayed" (John 9:3). Disease may also be God's means of taking His child home to heaven, or it can be supernaturally inflicted by Satan (e.g. the woman bent over for 18 years, Luke 13:11–16).

"The gifts of healings"

Upon Jesus' victorious return to heaven, there came to Christian believers an additional advantage. As was the custom of ancient rulers when they won battles over their enemies, they gave gifts to their subjects. So:

> When [Jesus] ascended on high,
>   he led captives in his train
>   and gave gifts to men. (Ephesians 4:8b)

These spiritual gifts are given according to the sovereign will of the Holy Spirit (1 Corinthians 12:11), and are listed in three gift lists (Romans 12:6–8; 1 Corinthians 12:8–10 and 28–30; Ephesians 4:8–11). Included are "the gifts of healings" (1 Corinthians 12:9, 28, literal translation). Most Bible scholars interpret the double plural, "gifts of healings" in one of four ways:

1. Holistic healing in the realm of the physical, emotional and spiritual are all possibilities.

2. Each healing in itself is a gift of God.

3. There are various forms of the gift for various illnesses.

4. No one person has a "gift of healing" as he or she might have a gift of prophecy or a gift of administration. For example, although healings took place through the ministries of Peter and Paul, they did not claim to have the gift of healing.

The "gifts of healings" were given by the risen, ascended, victorious Jesus to the local church and depend upon the Holy Spirit's sovereign will for the decisions and power to heal (1 Corinthians 12:6). The church has this added blessing beyond medical science.

How should the local church take advantage of the "gifts of healings"? It would appear that the normal use of the gifts of healings would be by the church elders' anointing the sick with oil (James 5:14–16) and offering believing prayer for the total restoration of those who are suffering.

Heart-Talk

Emotionally (I feel): I feel numb inside from the final diagnosis that I definitely have cancer. I am feeling weary from the tests and emotionally drained.

Intellectually (I think): I will meditate upon these healing promises in the Bible:

> I am the Lord, who heals you.
>   (Exodus 15:26)

> Praise the Lord, O my soul,
>   and forget not all his benefits—
> who forgives all your sins
>   and heals all your diseases.
>   (Psalm 103:2–3)

> Jesus answered them, "It is not the healthy who need a doctor, but the sick."
>   (Luke 5:31)

> This is the confidence we have in approaching God: that if we ask anything according to his will, he hears us.
>   (1 John 5:14)

Volitionally (I choose): I believe that Jesus, in His death on the cross, provided divine healing for both sin and sickness. I will allow His supernatural power to supplement the doctors' treatments. I will take advantage of the "gifts of healings" in the local church.

Prayer

Dear Heavenly Father, I praise You for Your benefits of forgiveness and healing. I thank You for my oncologist with his or her training in medical science. I recognize that You use doctors who practice medicine and surgery, but You are the Great Physician, and in the final analysis, You do the healing. I believe that You can perform miracles. I commit myself—body, soul and spirit—to You to heal in any manner You wish. In Jesus' name, amen.

"I pick James's prescription administered by the elders of the local church, then leave the healing results to God."

Is any one of you sick? He should call the elders of the church to pray over him and anoint him with oil in the name of the Lord. And the prayer offered in faith will make the sick person well; the Lord will raise him up. If he has sinned, he will be forgiven.
James 5:14–15

How often has it happened and still does, that devils have been driven out in the name of Christ, also by calling on His name and prayer that the sick have been healed.
Martin Luther

One evening, following my diagnosis of lymphoma in the advanced stage, I experienced an emotional letdown. It was that evening that our church elder, Rev. Harold May, and two other church leaders came into my hospital room to anoint me with oil and to pray for me. My wife, Elaine, and our two sons, Stephen and David, were already there. What more could a cancer patient ask for during so crucial a time? I had the support of my family and the spiritual support of my church.

Brother May, as we affectionately called him, was at the time well into his 80s. A retired pastor, he was one of the most gifted, creative and godly elders I have ever known. He had a kind and gentle heart that was as large as his huge frame. We spent a good time of fellowship together there in the hospital room. Then I shared with the men my thorough personal heart examination and how the Lord had reminded me of my mid-life verse.

Brother May said, "I feel a great spiritual struggle going on concerning your cancer. Let us believe God together to heal you." Opening a small vial of oil, he put some on the tip of his index finger and with it touched my forehead. Then, placing his huge hand on my head, he prayed with great compassion and zeal that the Lord would show mercy on me with His healing power. He rebuked Satan and prayed that I would be loosed from this cancer.

Brother May was an old-fashioned, no-nonsense, Bible-believing preacher who was convinced that the devil was the culprit in all sin, sickness and misery in the world. When he prayed, it was with the realization that spiritual warfare has been going on since Adam and Eve sinned in the Garden. He waged his attack against the enemy of my soul. He reminded the devil of his defeat by Jesus on the cross. He claimed healing for me in the powerful name of Jesus.

We all responded with a hearty "Amen!" I felt the weight lift from my heart. That evening my faith put on wings as I experienced the presence of Christ.

Jesus left His legacy of healing to the local church

Since that evening, I can identify with the cancer patient whose hope rises when supported by his or her local church in obedience to the prescription given by James (5:13–16). Jesus left His legacy of healing to the church together with the procedure to tap into His restorative power. To me, this procedure is one of the great wonders that many local churches need to recover in ministering to victims of cancer and all other forms of illness.

James, the faithful pastor, and his elders were carrying on through the "gifts of healings" the legacy given by the Holy Spirit to the church. A study of church history shows that whenever it has been faithful in following the procedure outlined by James, healings have resulted.

One of the greatest needs of the cancer patient is the church's spiritual support system that offers James's prescription for holistic healing. James prescribes (1) prayer, (2) faith and (3) confession as the spiritual medicine for wholeness.

The element of prayer

The key words *pray* and *prayer* are found five times in James 5:13–16. The church forms a support system of prayer that is vital to the health of every believer. The local church has been ordered by the Lord to get involved in the healing ministry through a specific course of action. This action begins with prayer. Suffering and sickness in the life of a fellow Christian are the signals for the church to pray.

Three classes in the church are responsible to pray. First, the one who is sick is encouraged to pray: "Let him pray" (5:13). It may be difficult to pray after the shocking pronouncement of cancer, for the patient is generally stunned by disbelief and denial of the disease. However, the prayer need not be lengthy. Peter, as he was beginning to sink in the stormy sea, prayed just three words: "Lord, save me!" (Matthew 14:30). Such a short but powerful prayer can keep a person from sinking into gloom. It allows the Lord to minister to damaged emotions.

The second group responsible to pray is the body of elders. "[The sick person] should call the elders of the church to pray over him" (5:14). Why are the local church elders singled out to pray for the sick? They are the spiritual leaders of the local church. Who would be better qualified than these who represent maturity, faith and spirituality? James himself was an excellent model of the church elder who spends much time in prayer. Tradition says he was nicknamed Camel Knees because of the callouses that developed from his hours of kneeling in prayer.

The third group called to prayer is the local church body as a whole: "Pray for each other so that you may be healed" (5:16). A cancer patient who knows his fellow church members are supporting him through prayer receives hope and encouragement to battle against the disease.

My cousin David, a young man in his 20s dying of leukemia, could not bear the sickening effects of the treatments. He was about to give up hope. But David was told that his church was praying for him. That assurance gave David faith to cope with the treatments, and he survived. Today he is strong and healthy. For the past 20 years he has lived a normal life.

The prescription of faith

Few concepts in the Bible are as important as faith. Faith is seen in every aspect of our relationship with God. Hal Lindsey lists some vital aspects of the Christian life that come by faith:

> We are born into eternal life through faith; we are declared righteous before God by

faith; we are forgiven by faith; we are healed by faith; we learn God's Word by faith; by faith we understand things to come; we walk by faith and not by sight; we overcome the world by faith; we enter God's rest by faith and we are controlled and empowered by the Holy Spirit by faith. We can only please God by faith, and everything we seek to do for God that is not from the source of faith is sin.[1]

James couples faith with prayer: "The prayer offered in faith will make the sick person well; the Lord will raise him up" (5:15). In understanding the "prayer offered in faith," we may find it helpful to consider what the prayer offered in faith is *not*.

For some time doctors have known that some patients respond to placebos—medications prescribed more for the patient's mental relief than for any actual effect on the disorder. The person takes the medication with the high hope that it will cure the problem at hand—and promptly begins to feel better.

I saw an article in our local newspaper reporting that some people believe crystal rocks have healing powers. These people spend time meditating in a quiet room, holding a whitish-pink chunk of quartz. They believe this helps to eliminate negative attitudes and stress. It helps, they say, "to achieve inner balance and to increase personal awareness." For them, crystals link ancient beliefs by the Mayans, Tibetans, Incas and American Indians, who used crystal rocks for healing and sacred ceremonies.[2]

In these two examples, faith is resting in either pills or rocks. They have made up their minds that what they want they will receive— faith on demand, as some have termed it. This misconception of biblical faith is self-centered, not Christ-centered.

The prayer of faith is Christ-centered

The healing benefits of the church rest in Christ-centered praying. Jesus Christ, the Great Physician, is central whenever heads are bowed in prayer for one who is sick. Biblical faith originates, takes root, grows and matures through the Word of God. "Faith comes from hearing the message, and the message is heard through the word of Christ" (Romans 10:17). God's final word is revealed in His Son:

> In the past God spoke to our forefathers through the prophets at many times and in various ways, but in these last days he has spoken to us by his Son, whom he appointed heir of all things, and through whom he made the universe. The Son is the radiance of God's glory and the exact representation of his being, sustaining all things by his powerful word. (Hebrews 1:1–3a)

The prayer of faith is our response to the revealed Word of God. The object of our faith is Jesus, the Creator of the universe, the Radiance of God's glory and the Sustainer of all things "by his powerful word." The prayer of faith lets go of selfish demands and submits to the Lordship of Jesus Christ. The One who made the universe and sustains all things by His Word is the Head of the Church. The local church is the instrument of the living Christ, who is the same yesterday, today and forever.

Why is oil combined with the prayer of faith? Because oil is symbolic of the Holy Spirit. It is the responsibility and ministry of the Holy Spirit to glorify Jesus and guide us into all truth (John 16:13–14), including the truth of divine healing. Oil centers the attention on Jesus Christ. He Himself is at the center of the healing ministry of the Church. When the sufferer is anointed with oil, all the focus of the elders and the patient is concentrated on the Lord Jesus Christ. Oil is an encouragement to faith. It is important to note that the prayer, not the oil, is the means of healing. When we lose sight of the focal point of faith in Christ, we are no longer resting in the revealed Word of God. Thus, if the will of God is healing for a cancer patient, the Spirit-filled elders will be given the prayer of faith for that healing. If it is not in the will of God, we have been obedient to the model of James and must leave the results with God.

There is instruction in the well-known incident of the paralyzed man brought to Jesus by some of his friends:

> Some men brought [Jesus] a paralytic, lying on a mat. When Jesus saw their faith, he said to the paralytic, "Take heart, son; your sins are forgiven."
>
> At this, some of the teachers of the law said to themselves, "This fellow is blaspheming!"
>
> Knowing their thoughts, Jesus said, "Why do you entertain evil thoughts in your hearts? Which is easier: to say, 'Your sins are forgiven,' or to say, 'Get up and walk'? But so that you may know that the Son of Man has authority on earth to forgive sins. . . ." Then he said to the paralytic, "Get up, take your mat and go home." And the man got up and went home. (Matthew 9:2–8)

Note two essential elements in this account. First the priority of spiritual healing. This is consistent with God's Word. The paralyzed man's soul was cleansed of sin and then his body was healed. It is significant that Jesus commanded, "Take heart, son; your sins are forgiven." Jesus started from the inside, with his heart, and worked outward to his body. Spiritual healing is essential for the healing of the body. Dr. A.Z. Hall, a medical doctor and former medical missionary, has noted:

> His body might have been healed, might have become a perfect instrument, but an instrument for what? Mind and body might have become instruments of destruction. He had to be cleansed and made fit for the Master's use.[3]

The second important element is the combined faith of the paralytic's friends: "When Jesus saw their faith." They formed the support system of faith in the healing power of Jesus. These true friends saw the miracles Jesus had performed and they carried their paralyzed friend to Him. Jesus rewarded their faith by healing the man of both sin and sickness. This illustrates the power of a support group such as the local church.

The threefold prescription of prayer, faith and confession of sin is the spiritual preparation needed for holistic healing. When we practice this procedure we please the Great Physician and leave the healing results to Him.

Perhaps physical healing will not occur, as was the case with Paul and his "thorn in the flesh" (2 Corinthians 12:7) or Trophimus's sickness (2 Timothy 4:20). They had, however, spiritual health, and that is of far greater value than physical healing.

Paul could have permitted his handicap to interrupt his evangelistic, missionary ministry. He could have pitied himself and said, "This is the end of my ministry of healing. How can I preach and teach healing unless God heals me personally?" But Jesus said to Paul, "My grace is sufficient for you, for my power is made perfect in weakness" (2 Corinthians 12:9). Out of his humility Paul wrote, "May I never boast except in the cross of our Lord Jesus Christ, through which the world has been crucified to me, and I to the world" (Galatians 6:14).

The prescription of confessing sin

A confessing church is a spiritually healthy church. This speaks of spiritual openness, which sets the climate for cleansing and healing. Cleansing and healing go together in that order. Confession is necessary for at least three reasons:

1. Sickness began as a result of the curse of sin. When we go to the doctor for treatment, the doctor diagnoses the disease and prescribes a remedy. James diagnosed the first cause as sin. This does not mean, of course, that the sick person or the cancer patient is a greater sinner than a healthy person.

2. Sin must be removed, for it is an obstacle to healing. Sin's removal allows the Holy Spirit to probe the heart when the patient is searching out any spiritual causes of his or her sickness as well as confessing any present sins.

3. Sin is an obstacle to the prayer of faith.

Unconfessed sin hardens the heart and results in unbelief. Unconfessed sin remains a barrier to faith.

The whole support group needs to make confession. Bill Gothard presents this insight:

> It is in this context of prayer that sins are to be confessed and forsaken both in the lives of the elders as well as in the life of the one who is sick. In order to identify sin, the elders must have spiritual perception in understanding cause-effect sequences.[4]

The healing support model in James

Listed in the diagram on the next page are the steps for the cancer patient to follow and the counsel for the support group to give. What more can we do than to follow James's prescription? God does heal through miraculous intervention in keeping with His own sovereign purposes. He also withholds healing, but this should not discourage us, for He answers prayer in ways that will amaze us. All that God requires of us is to focus on Jesus and His revealed Word and to leave the results with Him.

The highest kind of faith

That night in the hospital room, as I followed James's prescription, I had high hopes of

Cancer Patient	*Counsel of Support Group*
1. Personal prayer.	
2. Ask for help from elders.	Elders meet with the patient at a convenient place and hour.
3. Humbly admit cancer. "I'm scared and depressed. I feel very helpless."	Listen and empathize. Allow pain to be expressed. Pray. Share James's prescription.
4. Remove hindrances. Confess sins of the mind, emotions and will: impure thought life, negative emotions and sinful actions.	Confess own sins that would hinder the prayer of faith. Give scriptural solutions to spiritual problems. Replace evil with good.
5. Pray.	Annoint with oil. Pray in faith.
6. Leave the results—cleansing, forgiveness and healing—to God.	Assure the patient of continued support.

receiving immediate healing. It did not happen. In my case, healing would take time. When and how healing occurs is entirely in the hands of God. The healing may not take place until the completed healing at the resurrection of the body. When visible results do not immediately occur, Christians often feel guilty. They believe they did not exercise enough faith. It is possible, however, that they may be exercising a higher level of faith when they do not see the miraculous intervention of God in physical healing.

The highest kind of faith is modeled in Hebrews 11. The whole chapter describes what was accomplished by the faith of specific Old Testament heroes. The faith of those first mentioned often led to miraculous deliverances. The writer refers to those

> . . . who through faith conquered kingdoms, administered justice, and gained what was promised; who shut the mouths of lions, quenched the fury of the flames, and escaped the edge of the sword; whose weakness was turned to strength; and who became powerful in battle and routed foreign armies. Women received back their dead, raised to life again. (Hebrews 11:33–35a)

But the writer mentions a second group. This group experienced no miracles, no deliverances.

> Others were tortured and refused to be released, so that they might gain a better resurrection. Some faced jeers and flogging, while still others were chained and put in prison. They were stoned; they were sawed in two; they were put to death by the sword. They went about in sheepskins

and goatskins, destitute, persecuted and mistreated. (Hebrews 11:35b–37)

This second group demonstrated an even higher kind of faith. When no miracle happened, it meant their trials were not removed. Thus, faith had to continue amid the testing. It must have required a tremendous amount of faith to go through those difficult trials when there was no miraculous deliverance. Jesus said, "Blessed are those who have not seen and yet have believed" (John 20:29b).

Old Testament Job is another example of one who trusted God when he saw no evidence of deliverance. He cried out, "Though [God] slay me, yet will I hope in Him" (Job 13:15a). This is the highest kind of faith. Job did not say, "If I hope in God, He will not slay me." He said, "If God slays me, I will still hope in Him; I will still trust Him." Dr. Maurice R. Irvin wrote of this highest kind of trust:

> The person who remains unalterably committed to God and unfalteringly consistent in his service to the Lord need feel no guilt nor embarrassment. He is exercising far more faith than the person who believes in God because of what he can see.[5]

Heart-Talk

Emotionally (I feel): I feel lonely and need a supportive church, family and friends. My body and emotions are in bad shape. Gloomy thoughts of needles, chemo and pain make me feel anxious. I am struggling with negative feelings that seem to overwhelm my faith for healing.

Intellectually (I think): I am filling my mind with and meditating on these healing verses:

> He who conceals his sins does not prosper,
>   but whoever confesses and renounces them finds mercy. (Proverbs 28:13)

> Everyone born of God overcomes the world. This is the victory that has overcome the world, even our faith. (1 John 5:4)

> The prayer offered in faith will make the sick person well; the Lord will raise him up. If he has sinned, he will be forgiven. (James 5:15)

> Stretch out your hand to heal and perform miraculous signs and wonders through the name of your holy servant Jesus. (Acts 4:30)

Volitionally (I choose): I choose to call the elders to anoint me with oil and pray for me. I will follow James's threefold prescription. I will focus on Jesus and will not make any selfish "faith-on-demand" prayers. I will follow the counsel given by the elders and will agree with them for whatever healing Jesus has for me.

Prayer

Dear Heavenly Father, I marvel at the prescription of faith, prayer and confession of sin that prepares me for the results of Your healing power. Help me to focus my faith on Jesus. May I be willing to cooperate with the elders as they counsel me. Help me to be open and honest in my confession. I believe that You can heal me. I leave the healing results with You. In Jesus' name, amen.

"If I select the wonders of modern medicine, I must be prepared to manage the not-so-wonderful side effects."

On hearing this, Jesus said, "It is not the healthy who need a doctor, but the sick."
Matthew 9:12

The power of science to affect the way the body feels and functions is accelerating so fast that medical knowledge is said to double every five years. [1] U.S. News and World Report

Until recently, medical science has made slow, steady progress since Hippocrates, the father of medicine, treated patients in 400 B.C. with barley soup called *ptisan* and an extract of vinegar and honey. In our generation, however, there have been explosive advances in nearly every area of medicine.

Several years ago *Family Circle* magazine selected a panel of 17 top medical experts and asked their predictions concerning the advances we can anticipate within the next half century. This assembly of medical practitioners, researchers, educators and administrators were upbeat concerning the future. The magazine summarized their conclusions this way:

> By the year 2032 many cancers will be cured, artificial hearts will be "routine" and medical science will even prevent some mental illnesses. Best of all, *Family Circle* super-specialists predict that Americans will live 80 to 90 good years.[2]

Motivated by the U.S. government's "War on Cancer" declared in 1970, researchers have been testing anticancer drugs with a passion never known in this field. It is estimated that "over half a million chemicals have been screened for antitumor activity. Over 40 drugs have undergone trials, resulting in more than a dozen . . . now used frequently."[3]

Managing the side effects of modern medicine

The rapid advance of medical technology has produced many side effects for both the medical profession and its patients. It is helpful for both the profession and the patients to recognize at least four unpleasant side effects and to prepare to manage them with wisdom.

First is the unpleasant side effect of outdated

techniques and facilities. With medical knowledge doubling every five years, both textbooks and techniques frequently are out of date. Administrators of continuing education programs have their work cut out for them. So does the medical profession generally, if it is to keep current.

I am grateful that, in the sovereignty of God, I was near the University of Michigan Hospital. This hospital is a pioneer in treating lymphoma and has remained on the cutting edge when it comes to that disease. At the time I was there, however, the university was constructing a new medical building to house its state-of-the-art equipment. Temporarily they had to place their CAT Scanner in inadequate space.

On the day of my test, the first order of business was for me to drink a bottle-full of unidentified purple liquid. Then the technician instructed me to lie down on a bedlike slab that ran on a track into the center of the large donut-shaped machine. He placed both of my arms over my head, attaching one to an IV needle. We were ready for business.

As the machine went leisurely about its picture taking, I could feel the effects of that bottle of purple beginning to build in my bladder. Finally, I became terribly uncomfortable.

"Are you almost finished?" I shouted to the technician who was in a glass-encased control room.

He assured me he was almost finished. The machine continued to take pictures. I waited and waited in increasing desperation.

"I'm about to burst!" I finally said. "Is there a restroom in here I can use the moment you are finished?"

"There is no restroom," the technician answered. "There was not enough room in here for both the equipment and a restroom."

Can you imagine! I thought to myself. *A million dollar piece of equipment and no restroom!*

A second unpleasant side effect of our high tech generation is the moving from friendly family doctor to the unfeeling specialist. Unfortunately, technological advances have caused these medical specialists to treat patients like machines rather than people. In his book *Healing and the Scriptures*, the late D. Martyn Lloyd-Jones, noted English pastor and himself a medical doctor, has a chapter entitled "Medicine in Modern Society," based on his lectures to members of the Christian Medical Fellowship, the British Medical Association and the Royal Commonwealth Society. He says to doctors:

> Do unto others what you would have others do unto you. It is a very good test. . . . Would you like to have this catheter pushed down your veins and into your heart? Would you like it to be done to you?

Above all, be concerned for people as people. Be concerned for the whole man. Never was there greater need for character in medical men—understanding, sympathy and patience. Yes, and self-sacrifice.[4]

A third unpleasant side effect for both hospitals and patients is the skyrocketing costs of modern medicine. Having a limited amount of hospitalization is an added burden. Struggling to pay medical expenses can be a never-ending problem.

In the days of Jesus, doctors were few. Their skills were limited and no doubt expensive. This is implied in the account of the woman whom Jesus healed of her bleeding. Prior to her healing, Luke, the physician, describes her this way:

A woman was there who had been subject to bleeding for twelve years, but no one could heal her. (Luke 8:43)

But Mark, who was *not* a doctor, minces no words to describe the woman's plight:

A woman was there who had been subject to bleeding for twelve years. She had suffered a great deal under the care of many doctors and had spent all she had, yet instead of getting better she grew worse. (Mark 5:25–26)

Can you see this pathetic, desperate woman going from one doctor to another for 12 long years? Each one held out hope to her. Each, in return for his fee, delivered disappointment. But whatever the fees that had impoverished this woman, they could not begin to compare with today's astronomical medical expenses.

The fourth unpleasant side effect is the host of legal, ethical and religious questions complex enough to tax the wisdom of Solomon. Making the decision to undergo chemotherapy is not easy. Basically, it boils down to an ethical and a religious question. Is the uncertain prognosis of full recovery worth exposing one's body to a treatment that can have severe emotional and physical outcome? If this human body is the temple of the Holy Spirit, is it right to allow a powerful poison to be injected into it? The body's immune system has been God-given to protect against disease. Each injection of chemo temporarily destroys the immune system, opening the body to risk of outside infection. Added to this is the body's greatly lessened ability to coagulate blood. Severe bleeding could result.

A television series on the Public Broadcasting Network, "Managing Our Miracles," demonstrated the complex legal, ethical and religious issues raised by the modern miracles of medicine. The program centered around a panel of health experts, including former Surgeon General C. Everett Koop and other noted doctors, nurses, clergy and lawyers. The panel was presented with classic case studies arising out of modern medical practice. The varied responses clearly indicated how frequently decisions become entangled in legal and ethical issues.

One example was the much-publicized case of William Schroeder, in 1986 the longest surviving artificial heart recipient. More than a year had passed since his seemingly successful operation, but three strokes had left him weak and unable to speak.

"I wish Bill had written down on the consent form at what point he would want to say, 'Stop this; I've had enough,' " said Schroeder's wife, Margaret. But Bill made no such comment.

Should Bill have been allowed to die? Why? Why not? Who should decide? Why? Are people playing God if they "pull the plug"? How would you feel if you had been Bill? Margaret? The children? Bill's doctor?

Prolonged life or extended dying?

Dr. Rob Ray MacGregor, professor of medicine and chief of the infectious disease section at the University of Pennsylvania School of Medicine, believes that "medical care, American style, is clearly running the risk of extending the dying process rather than prolonging life":

Because of powerful tools at our disposal,

we doctors sometimes abdicate our tradi-
tional role as a servant and advisor to the
sick and suffering and become technicians
who merely run the machines that sustain
life (defined in a narrow physiological
sense). . . .

Is respiration failing? Use the respirator.
Have the kidneys stopped working? Start
dialysis. Slowly and sadly our attitude is
becoming: "If we have the technical
capability, we must always use it." And as
a result, patients can be drawn into a
dehumanizing spiral in which each organ
failure is met by still another life-support
procedure.[5]

When to "pull the plug"

MacGregor, writing in *Christianity Today*, sets
out five biblical principles for the sustain-
life/let-die debate. I have somewhat condensed
them.[6]

1. The overriding teaching of the New
Testament is love. . . . What is the loving
thing to do in this circumstance? Is it
loving to maintain hope when realistically
there is none?

2. "Always treat others as you would like
them to treat you" (Matthew 7:12 NEB). .
. . It may be surprising to learn that many
doctors share the average layman's fear of

a lingering death and instruct their families that they want no "heroic measures" to be used when their time comes.

3. Scripture teaches that love between God and man is "better than life" (Psalm 63:3). Thus, God does not tell us that earthly life is to be valued as the highest good, nor have the apostles, martyrs and saints lived this way through the centuries. Paul said: "For to me, to live is Christ and to die is gain" (Philippians 1:21).

4. "Man is destined to die once, and after that to face judgment" (Hebrews 9:27) is a reminder to modern medicine that normally people prepare "to die once." However, when trying to do all we can for the dying patient, we put many through a psycho-physiological tug-of-war with death because our technological interventions repeatedly "rescue" the patient from the inevitability of death.

5. "You will know the truth, and the truth will set you free" (John 8:32) seems to be applicable. The truth can set one free both from false guilt and from the need to use unwarranted therapeutic maneuvers. Appropriate care balances a respect for the process of dying. The physician and family can elect to make a patient comfortable without resorting to costly procedures that prove in the end to be fruitless and punishing. . . . Our own personal walk with

Christ and the support of the fellowship of believers can empower us to emulate His compassion rather than be driven by the technological imperative.

Such decisions are never easy. They require God's guidance.

"The End Is Not the End"

This touching testimony by C. Everett Koop, also appeared in *Christianity Today*:

My mother was 87 when she died of uterine cancer. She was in a coma, during which people actually asked me if I wanted to put her on dialysis. That would have been ridiculous for personal, spiritual and economic reasons.

I do not believe—and have never taught—that every patient should be kept alive for the longest time possible. Nor have I said every patient has to have the last bit of high-tech heroic treatment available. I do believe in the right of the patient to say, 'I have lived my life,' and to choose his or her own treatment. But that question becomes complicated when we consider the decisions people make for others who are not cognitive and have not made their final wishes known.

Right now, I am 70 years old and in excellent health. If my kidneys shut down tomorrow, let us say, after a severe infection, I don't know how long I would want to be on dialysis. It would be foolish and a waste of resources for me to have a kidney transplant at my age. I would probably opt to clean up my affairs, say goodbye to my family and drift out in uremia.

The important point is that my wife and I know exactly how each of us feels about the end of life. This will be crucial if the time comes to make such a decision and I'm not then able to do so. Of course, all such talk has different connotations for the Christian than for the non-Christian. My wife knows I do not believe in being ushered out of this life with a lethal injection. I want to hang around long enough to be sure my family is taken care of. But after that, I don't want my life prolonged in great discomfort when it is fruitless.

I don't look forward to the manner in which I am going to die. But I do not fear death. Indeed, the way in which we face death is a matter of faith. For the Christian, it is not the end.[7]

"Till Death Do Us Part"

Edith Schaeffer, widow of the late apologist Francis Schaeffer, recounts his final days, giving a beautiful model of a Christian couple creatively preparing for death:

Fran came across the Atlantic Ocean from L'Abri, Switzerland, in December, 1983, for cancer treatment at the Mayo Clinic in Rochester, Minnesota. He was very ill, and the flight was a difficult one. On the way from the airport to the hospital, the doctors in the ambulance were reporting by walkie-talkie his pulse beat, blood pressure and rate of breathing, all of which were rather alarming. When we finally got to the hospital, a doctor told me he doubted Fran would live through the night. I told him I would call upon God and ask Him to be the one to make that judgment.

The next morning, Fran was better. He opened his eyes and said to me, "Edith, would you be willing to buy a house near the hospital so I don't ever have to cross the ocean again and so I could go home and have my things around me?" Of course I said I would, believing that was part of what I had promised in my marriage vows when I said, "For better or for worse . . . till death do us part."

That evening, I passed a house with a "For Sale" sign in the lawn, and within a week I was signing the papers. A month later, I was back at L'Abri, packing all the possessions of our married life into 269 boxes. It was another five weeks until those boxes reached Rochester. During that time, Fran was in and out of the hospital and on two speaking tours. He was only in the newly furnished house two days before he returned to the hospital for the last time.

On Easter Day, six doctors called me into a room, and the leading consultant said, "He is dying of cancer. Do you want him placed in intensive care on machines? Once a person is on machines, I would never pull the plug. I need to know what your viewpoint is."

Many thoughts went through my head. I had for years talked with my husband about the preciousness of life, of the fact that even five minutes can make a difference if something needs to be said or needs to be done. We did not believe in putting a chain around our necks with a living will, because doctors and ambulance aides can make terrible mistakes. They could find that little tag and push the person aside and take care of someone else, when the one with the living will could have lived for another five years if given oxygen at the right time.

But there is no point in simply prolonging death. It is a fine line; it is not an absolute one-two-three process. There are differences from person to person, and it requires great wisdom.

Based on these thoughts, I told the doctor, "My feeling right now is that above all things, Fran wants to be with me. I haven't left him at all. I believe when my husband leaves his body, he will be with the Lord. I don't want him to leave me until he's with the Lord. Therefore, I am sure he would want to go to the house he asked me to buy and be there for the time he has left."

The doctors got the most relieved looks on their faces. One of them said, "I just wish more people would do things this way. That's the best kind of care at this time. That's the most helpful thing."

Soon Fran was home, in a bed facing four big panels of glass looking out on a deck with grass around it and trees with the first leaves of spring. The L'Abri workers went out and bought pots of geraniums so there would be an instant garden all around the window. All the things Fran loved in Switzerland were around him, just as he asked.

Music flooded the room. One after another, we played his favorite records: Beethoven, Bach, Schubert and Handel. Ten days later, on May 15, 1984, with the music of Handel's *Messiah* still in the air, Fran breathed his last breath.[8]

Heart-Talk

Emotionally (I feel): I dislike being in the hospital where I will be examined, tested, probed and pricked. I feel disoriented in this huge complex of mile-long corridors connecting rooms with patients, doctors, offices and equipment. I am uneasy when the doctor examines me, says little and leaves the room. I hurt and need a caring response.

Intellectually (I think): I am meditating on these encouraging promises:

> Cast all your anxiety on him because he cares for you. (1 Peter 5:7)

> When I am afraid,
>   I will trust in you.
> In God, whose word I praise,
>   in God I trust; I will not be afraid.
> What can mortal man do to me?
>   (Psalm 56:3–4)

> O Lord, you have searched me
>   and you know me.
> You know when I sit and when I rise;
>   you perceive my thoughts from afar. . . .
> For you created my inmost being;
>   you knit me together in my mother's
>   womb.
> I praise you because I am fearfully and
>   wonderfully made;
>   your works are wonderful,

I know that full well.
(Psalm 139:1–2, 13–14)

On hearing this, Jesus said, "It is not the healthy who need a doctor, but the sick." (Matthew 9:12)

Our dear friend Luke, the doctor, and Demas send greetings. (Colossians 4:14)

Volitionally (I choose): I choose to trust my doctor as the instrument of God's healing power and will take advantage of the best treatment and the latest technology. All my cares, from finances to dying gracefully, I cast upon the Lord. I trust Him to keep me from the serious side effects of modern medicine. I will inform my family not to permit any "heroic" measures should I become mentally incompetent.

Prayer

Dear Heavenly Father, I thank You for the wonder of modern medicine that in Your divine providence has given me a greater hope of survival. I pray for Your strength to overcome the unpleasant side effects of modern medicine. May my oncologist and the other doctors and nurses show kindness and treat me as a person. Help me not to complain. I pray You will guide the doctors and medical staff in the healing process. In Jesus' name, amen.

"I practice positional thinking that produces power to live above tough circumstances."

And God raised us up with Christ and seated
us with him in the heavenly realms in Christ
Jesus. Ephesians 2:6

In contrast to the popular exhortation to
"keep looking up" (from ourselves to Christ),
we are to "keep looking down" (from our position in Him) upon our circumstances here on
earth.[1] Miles J. Stanford

When entering the world of cancer, a person quickly realizes that pain occupies
more than just the physical realm. Pain affects
the whole person. Each part of the whole has a
potential for suffering, and each part affects
the whole person. We are open to damage or
loss spiritually, emotionally, physically and so-
cially.

Study the lists on the next page to be aware
of a sampling of the potential damage cancer

may trigger in a person's life. The world of cancer is like a shower of arrows that rain upon the whole person. And when it rains it pours. We are amazed at the wonders of modern medicine with its advanced knowledge and technology. But there will be pain because we are human. The body is not like an insensitive automobile that a mechanic can repair. The human body is one part of a complex person composed also of soul and spirit. All three react together to pain.

Potential for Damage and Pain in the World of Cancer

Spiritual Damage

Prayerlessness
Insecurity
Guilt
God seems far away
Hopelessness
"Why me, God?"
Unbelief, doubt

Psychological Damage

Loss of control
Anxiety, worry
Fear of death
Fear of the future
Poor self-worth
Grief, depression
Bitterness

Social Damage

Loneliness
Isolation
Activities limited
Loss of job
Family trauma
Rejecting people
Cultural problems

Physical Damage

Loss of energy
Fever, sweats
Coughing
Weight loss
Violent nausea
Constipation
Bodily functions altered

When someone in pain from cancer arrives at the hospital, he or she realizes that it may require further pain to remove the growth that produced the original pain. The nurses cause pain as they inject needles to take blood. The oncologist, administering chemotherapy, exposes the patient to the extreme discomfort of nausea. My oncologist summed up the painful side effects of chemotherapy by saying, "I am going to make you very sick in order to make you well."

Much has been written on the value of positive thinking in overcoming hardship, disease and handicaps. There is growing evidence that a positive relationship between mind and body can influence the outcome of treatment. When we let ourselves indulge in negative responses such as anger, resentfulness and self-pity, these negative responses affect our bodies in ways that will hinder the healing process. They also hinder our spiritual growth. On the other hand, when we allow a positive outlook to fill our thinking, the healing process is more likely to take place.

Try the power of positional thinking

Jesus, through His death, has broken the power of the old nature in those of us who believe. By His resurrection He has raised us to an authoritative position in the heavenly realm. It is from that position that we have strength to battle the negative effects of cancer, wherever they attack. When our thinking is centered on Christ's death and resurrection, we have victory over our old nature.

Even though we have a new nature, it is still possible for us to let the old nature's thinking gain control of our mind. This becomes evident when we allow a whole flood of destructive emotions, as seen in the previous diagram, to influence us. Sometimes we gloss over our negative emotions; at other times family members try to protect us from them. We must expect emotional struggles. We must face them squarely. We must deal with them biblically for healing. How? Mary Beth Moster prescribed this helpful chart in her pocket guide, *When the Doctor Says It's Cancer:*[2]

> If we confess our sins, he is faithful and just and will forgive us our sins and purify us from all unrighteouness. 1 John 1:9

We who have experienced cancer understand

Facing a Negative Emotion

1. Identify it.
2. Acknowledge it.
3. See it as God sees it.
4. When it is sin, confess it.
5. Ask God to replace it with a positive emotion.

---

the battle between our two inner natures that can bring out our worst sides. What we think about turns out to be a reflection of either our old nature or our new nature. How do we respond when our old nature asserts itself? We can creatively cope as we center our thoughts on our twofold death/resurrection position with Christ.

Identified with Christ's death and resurrection

As we saw earlier, Jesus in His death and resurrection identified with us. It follows, therefore, that as believers we were identified with Him in both His death and resurrection. This being so:

1. *We must think co-crucifixionally:* the old life is dead and buried. Our old selves died and were buried with Jesus when He died and was buried. The power of the old nature has been broken. We need to think of the old life as dead and buried; this forms the "death position." Whenever a negative emotion such as depression enters our hearts to take control, think position. We do not respond to these negative emotions as we did when we lived under the control of our sinful natures. In our new position, we have Christ's power to respond to destructive emotions in a positive way. Our old selves were crucified once for all on the cross. They are, in fact, buried with Christ. Paul tes-

tified of his co-crucifixion with Christ when he declared:

> I have been crucified with Christ and I no longer live, but Christ lives in me. The life I live in the body, I live by faith in the Son of God, who loved me and gave himself for me. (Galatians 2:20)

2. *We must also think co-resurrectionally:* the new life is in heaven with Jesus. The Bible says:

> [God] raised [Jesus] from the dead and seated him at his right hand in the heavenly realms. (Ephesians 1:20)

> God raised us up with Christ and seated us with him in the heavenly realms in Christ Jesus. (Ephesians 2:6)

Our new nature is alive. By faith it has been raised with Christ and has ascended with Him into heaven. Through His death, resurrection and ascension, Jesus Christ has put us in this new exalted position. Thus, when negative emotions such as a spirit of depression try to gain control, we must not only think the "death position" to the old nature but also the "risen life position" of the new nature. Look at the following diagram to grasp this twofold position:

Death Position	Life Position
If we died with Christ. . .	. . . we will also live with him. Romans 6:8
united in his death. . .	. . . united in his ressurection. Romans 6:5
I have been crucified . . .	. . . I live by faith. Galatians 2:20
For you died . . .	. . . your life is now hidden with Christ. Colossians 3:3

A pastor, making a hospital call on one of the members of his congregation, asked, "How are you doing?"

"Under these circumstances," replied the patient, "not very well."

"That is your main problem," the pastor quickly answered. "As a Christian, you should be living *above* your circumstances, not under them."

I thank the Lord for this "positional" truth that strengthened me to cope with the spiritual, psychological and social damages of cancer. I also thank Him for His daily healing touches to my body. How did I practice the power of positional thinking? By beginning the morning with prayer. Part of that prayer was this: "Lord Jesus, thank You for Your death and resurrection for me. I count my old self to be dead with Your death and my new self to be alive through Your resurrection. As I take my seat with You in the heavenlies, I claim Your resurrection power for this day."

Whenever I experienced an unusual amount of physical pain, such as the "night sweats" or the bouts of violent nausea, my prayer would be, "Lord Jesus, I take Your resurrection life for my body. May Your life flow through this body for a special quickening touch." On many such occasions, Elaine would be there to agree together with me in believing prayer for healing.

More than medicine at work during chemotherapy

After listening to the oncologist's explanation of chemotherapy and reading about it and its side effects, Elaine and I prayed for guidance. Was there a chance that it would arrest this fast-advancing cancer within me? Or was I simply postponing death a few weeks or months? After praying, both of us felt assured that God wanted us to proceed.

I signed the consent form.

Doctors began the program by injecting a bicarbonated solution intravenously. Due to my anemic condition, they added two units of blood while continuing the other solution. Later that afternoon, they appeared with a glass cylinder perhaps three inches long and the size of a half-dollar in diameter. In it was the anticancer drug, which they allowed to flow into a vein in the back of my hand. Only about

15 minutes elapsed before the contents emptied into my bloodstream. With this small dosage there were no side effects and no nausea. I praised the Lord.

That was Friday. On Sunday they discharged me from the hospital, scheduling X-rays for Tuesday. Months later they told me they had made an error in the initial chemo dosage. Instead of the comparatively small amount in the cylinder, I was to have received a massive initial dose. The bad news was that I had to take an extra treatment. The good news was that even with the mild dosage, the tumor pressing against the entry to one of the kidneys had in less than four days shrunk dramatically.

This latter report was the first good news we had received. Both Elaine and I were elated. For there to have been such a miraculous effect, more than medicine was at work. It was the beginning of many healing touches I experienced as I thought positionally, followed James's prescription and left the results with God.

Spiritual blessings begin in the heavenlies

Six months before doctors diagnosed my cancer, I had an unusual dream. I was walking on a path when darkness closed in on me. I found it more difficult to follow the path. The darkness overwhelmed me. I had a great sense of fear. Then, suddenly, a song came out of the darkness. I could hear both the melody and the lyrics repeated several times:

> All the time, any place,
>> I'll praise the Lord all the time,
>>> Praise Him.
>> Everywhere, all His grace,
>>> I'll praise the Lord all the time.

The darkness turned to light. Fear turned to joy. I awakened with a feeling of elation. Jumping out of bed, I grabbed a piece of paper and a pencil and hurried to the kitchen. While they were fresh in my mind, I jotted down the words and wrote the melody on a music staff.

In analyzing this unusual dream, I believe it was the result of a sermon I had preached the day before. My text was from Ephesians:

> Praise be to the God and Father of our Lord Jesus Christ, who has blessed us in the heavenly realms with every spiritual blessing in Christ. (1:3)

Evidently those words of the message had penetrated my subconscious mind and were released in the dream the following night. "Heavenly realms" is that spiritual sphere where we belong the moment we receive the miracle of spiritual life. Spiritual blessings originate in the heavenly realms.

With the sermon still fresh in my mind, I

went over the song again and asked myself the question, "Why can a Christian praise the Lord all the time?" The answer is in the same book of Ephesians:

> And God raised us up with Christ and seated us with him in the heavenly realms in Christ Jesus. (2:6)

We can praise the Lord all the time because we are seated in the heavenly realms. We are set free to live above the tough circumstances. The Lord replaces our negative emotions and spiritual depressions with His positive spiritual blessings. Thus, I added a stanza to the chorus of my dream:

> All the time, any place,
>   I'll praise the Lord all the time,
>   Praise Him.
> Everywhere, all His grace,
>   I'll praise the Lord all the time.
>
> I'm seated in the heavenlies,
>   Where spiritual blessings flow;
> My Father God gives them
>   For me to serve and to grow.

Little did I realize that I would soon be facing some of the darkest days I have ever experienced. I would be putting my faith on the line. Would I be prepared to rise above the circumstances "to serve" and "to grow"? Would I be willing to learn the lessons that I needed to learn to assist me in growing?

Positional thinking during the treatments

I received my chemotherapy treatments on an outpatient basis. I generally drove the 21 miles to the hospital. Elaine chauffeured me home because I was too ill to drive.

I shall never forget my first outpatient chemo session. Once we were at the hospital, X-rays and blood samples were routine procedures. They had to monitor my blood count to be sure my body could tolerate another treatment. I waited to be taken into one of the small treatment rooms. Nearby me a woman whom I judged to be in her 60s, sitting in a lounge chair, was receiving chemo from an IV bag on a pole next to her. I felt very apprehensive about the whole thing.

The nurse who administered the chemo was reassuring. She explained the procedures clearly. *If that 60-year-old woman can handle the treatment,* I thought, *I guess I can.* However, the woman became very nauseated toward the end, sending my emotions into a tailspin.

Help me to be level-headed and cool, dear Jesus, I prayed. *I claim Your promise, "I can do all things through [Christ] who gives me strength." I'm seated in heavenly places. I have the victory!*

About that time, a good looking 16-year-old boy entered the room. I learned that he was being treated for testicular cancer. I began to realize that in this frightening world of cancer, age and position mean nothing. Anger and compassion mixed within me at the sight of such a young person having to face the disease. I thanked the Lord for the good health of my two sons, Stephen and David. Even I had managed to escape cancer for 49 years. I was glad it was I and not Elaine or my sons who had the disease.

I smiled to myself. Already the "Why me?" question was turning to an acceptance of my affliction.

Now it was my turn. The nurse instructed me to place my arm on the arm rest, wrist down. Carefully she inserted the IV needle into a vein on the back of my hand and taped it in place. The combination of adriamyucin and vincristine began to flow.

I felt no ill effects until an hour after I arrived back home. Then nausea accompanied by vomiting overwhelmed me. For about six hours I vomited at 15-minute intervals. This was a foretaste of what would become routine after each treatment. Antinausea shots and pills had little effect on me.

God provides power to win, not to fail!

We are positionally in a place of strength. So why is it that many Christians who experience tragedies such as cancer have difficulty coping? The answer is clear. Many—even those who are thinking positively—are not thinking *positionally* in their everyday experiences. They are depending on themselves and their own human resources.

When it comes to coping with cancer, there are two mindsets:

Two Mindsets in Coping with Cancer

Positive thinking: *Based on the old nature*	*Positional thinking:* *Based on the new nature*
Self-centered	Christ-centered
Personal willpower	Christ's resurrection power
Earthly	Heavenly
Humanistic	Biblical
Dead to God	Alive to God
Self-glorifying	God-glorifying
Goal: self-realization	Goal: to know Christ

Not I, But Christ

Not I but Christ my every need supplying;
   Not I but Christ my strength and health
      to be;
Christ, only Christ for body, soul, and
      spirit;
   Christ, only Christ, live then Thy life in
      me.

Oh, to be saved from myself, dear Lord!
Oh, to be lost in Thee!
Oh, that it might be no more I,
But Christ that lives in me!
—Albert B. Simpson

The secret of positional victory

In the world of cancer, the drawing of blood becomes a necessary part of life and a dreaded routine. The week following each treatment I entered the outpatient section of our local hospital three successive days for the monitoring of the white cell and platelet counts. As the blood tests multiplied, my veins began to scar, making it difficult for blood to be drawn. In time several "pokes" became necessary to locate a "good spot." For these added anxious moments I relied on the strength of Christ through daily positional thinking.

The monitoring became a numbers game. It was necessary for the counts to return to normal levels before the next treatment. The hospital would phone the white and platelet counts to us. As the treatments progressed, the counts sunk to ever lower levels. My system had to work harder and harder to raise my blood count to an acceptable level for another dose of chemo.

Will the bone marrow be able to manufacture enough cells to bring the count back up to normal? I wondered. *Will my lowered white cell count still be able to fight infections?*

I felt very uncomfortable around people who sneezed or coughed. I withdrew from crowds as much as possible. I became almost paranoid about all the germs floating around me.

Another anxiety in the numbers game was the platelet count. Lower platelet counts decreased the ability of the blood to coagulate. *Will I bleed to death from a cut?* I asked myself.

The greatest help to counteract these anxious moments was positional thinking. I lived in constant fellowship with Jesus, who kept pouring His strength into me to stay on top of the numbers game. I learned how essential it is to live one day at a time. I did not have enough strength to cope with the next day's problems or to be overly concerned about the crises of the day before. But Jesus Christ strengthened me to meet the challenges confronting me that day.

Miles Stanford summarizes positional living with this slogan: *Abide above to grow below.*[3] He shares the following insight:

> When the Holy Spirit gives us adequate apprehension of our risen position, we are able spontaneously to reckon ourselves "alive unto God in Jesus Christ." Thus we are drawn to the source of our life, and there we learn to rest—and abide above![4]

My family and I praised the Lord when the blood counts began to rise again to normal levels. I appreciated the ability that our Creator God placed within my body to replenish cells that had been destroyed. God alone is independently self-sufficient. He created the human race to be dependent upon Him as the sovereign Lord of the universe. Jesus taught this dependency in the parable of the branch and the vine:

> I am the vine; you are the branches. If a man remains in me and I in him, he will bear much fruit; apart form me you can do nothing. (John 15:5)

On June 21, 1981, after the fifth chemotherapy treatment, I was examined by means of an ultrasound machine. "Please, Lord," I prayed, "may no cancer cells be found!" Later I received the results. The test was negative. Hallelujah! I was classified as "in remission."

Heart-Talk

Emotionally (I feel): I feel mental, emotional and physical pain throughout the chemo treatments. I fear that the chemo will not destroy all of the cancer. I dread the nausea that accompanies chemo and fear I will have serious side effects from the lowered white counts. The emotions of doubt, worry, anxiety, self-pity and depression are threatening to gain control of me.

Intellectually (I think): I am meditating on these healing verses:

> Since, then, you have been raised with Christ, set your hearts on things above, where Christ is seated at the right hand of God. Set your minds on things above, not on earthly things. For you died, and your life is now hidden with Christ in God. (Colossians 3:1–3)

> I pray also that the eyes of your heart may be enlightened in order that you may know the hope to which he has called you, the riches of his glorious inheritance in the saints, and his incomparably great power for us who believe. That power is like the working of his mighty strength, which he exerted in Christ when he raised him from the dead and seated him at his right hand in the heavenly realms, far above all rule and authority, power and dominion, and every title that can be given, not only in the present age but also in the one to come. (Ephesians 1:18–21)

Volitionally (I choose): I choose to practice the power of positional thinking and take my seat in the heavenly realms. I will depend on the power of the risen Savior to help me overcome all of the negative effects of cancer.

Prayer

Dear Heavenly Father, I praise Jesus for His death and resurrection that provide me with power to cope with cancer. Forgive me for the sin of negative thinking. I trust Your Holy Spirit to help me take my heavenly position upon rising each morning. I will live this new day in total dependence upon You. In Jesus' name, amen.

"When God withholds the miracle of instant healing, I humbly embrace His alternative of amazing grace that creates inner strength and a joyous disposition."

But he said to me, "My grace is sufficient for you, for my power is made perfect in weakness." Therefore I will boast all the more gladly about my weaknesses, so that Christ's power may rest on me. 2 Corinthians 12:9

He giveth more grace when
the burdens grow greater,
He sendeth more strength when
the labors increase;
To added affliction He addeth mercy,
To multiplied trials, His multiplied peace.[1]
Annie J. Flint

Grace expresses a marvelous and radical view of life different from any that could have been conceived by the human mind. Would you ever hear a nonchristian say, "My power to cope with cancer is strengthened and made perfect in weakness?" In contrast, you likely would hear the person say, "My power increases as I continue to think positively. I will not give up the fight. I can cope. I will overcome cancer." Although we laud those strong-willed individuals determined to overcome cancer through self-effort, they are not relying on the healing grace of God.

God's grace is another one of the great advantages the Christians have over nonchristians in coping with cancer. Grace gives us believers the power to creatively cope with the extreme pressures of suffering before, during and after the treatments. But grace does not merely provide a way to cope. It forces us to look beneath the surface of life in a way not otherwise possible and, as a result, to live life on a deeper level. It is essential, therefore, that we understand the meaning of grace and know how we may receive it to cope with suffering.

Five traits of grace

God's grace has five characterizing aspects.

1. *Grace reaches out to the whole human race.* Paul told Titus, "The grace of God that brings salvation has appeared to all men" (Titus 2:11). God takes the first step to extend His grace to a sinful and suffering humanity.

2. *Grace is free; it is not earned and it is not a*

reward for good performance. "It is by grace you have been saved through faith," Paul wrote to the Ephesians, "—and this not from yourselves, it is the gift of God—not by works, so that no one can boast" (Ephesians 2:8–9). Since God's unearned favor is freely given to us, it is foolish to try to "work for" free grace to gain salvation. Grace is also the basis for positional thinking, discussed in chapter 7. Just as we do not work for salvation, likewise we do not work for the inner power we already freely possess in the heavenly realms in Christ.

> It is by grace you have been saved. And God raised us up with Christ and seated us with him in the heavenly realms in Christ Jesus. (Ephesians 2:5–6)

3. *Grace grows when we live by it.* Peter admonishes those believers to whom he is writing to "grow in the grace and knowledge of our Lord and Savior Jesus Christ" (2 Peter 3:18). We are not only saved by grace but we are to live by grace. Unfortunately, when it comes to "living by grace," we sometimes substitute performance for grace. This is especially true of the cancer patient who allows cancer to make him or her feel worthless. This feeling is contrary to the wonder of grace.

It is useless to work for God's acceptance when we already possess it. Through grace we have God's unconditional love and total acceptance. It is an acceptance and a love that we did not earn. It was freely given to us in spite of our failures and sinful condition. Calvary demonstrates once and for all that we are not worthless.

We must not, therefore, allow cancer to breed in us feelings of worthlessness. We are of more value to God than all the combined wealth in the world. God put on flesh and died a cruel death in order to redeem us. This ought to convince us that, far from being worthless, we are to Him of great value. As we live in the strength of God's grace, it would be foolish to try to prove our worth by performance. As we rely on the power of grace and live by grace, we will grow in grace.

4. *Grace can be set aside or missed.* Paul said to the Galatians, "I do not set aside the grace of God" (Galatians 2:21a). The writer of Hebrews urged his readers, "See to it that no one misses the grace of God" (Hebrews 12:15a).

There are at least three ways to set aside or miss the grace of God. First, we can get caught up with "doing" rather than "being." We want to give the Lord some of our works while at the same time we hold onto ourselves. God wants us to surrender ourselves to Him so that He may develop our beings into Christlike character. His love is not based on what we do but on who He is. God is a loving Being who reaches out to us with unconditional love and sufficient grace to cope with all the suffering caused by cancer and its treatments.

Second, we miss grace or set it aside when we place value on our own strength and resources. Our culture dictates this kind of thinking. We have been conditioned to think "big," "fast," "successful." We can do and be anything we set our minds to. In a day of instant puddings, spray-on Band-Aids and microwave dinners, we want quick solutions to our problems. We want to get out from under the pressure of seemingly endless treatments. It takes time, however, for our Heavenly Father to discipline us. Those pressures we long to escape bring us to a deeper level of spiritual maturity than we could possibly achieve without them.

Third, we miss or set aside grace when we are not willing to let God teach us the greater spiritual realities that go deeper than our shallow living. Tim Hansel quotes Paul's accusation in Second Corinthians 10:7a—"You are only looking on the surface of things"—and gives us this insight into living by grace:

> Pain forces you to look below the surface. The tragedy is that many of us never have the courage to choose to do that. Hence we waste much of our life in bitterness and complaint, always looking for something else, never realizing that perhaps God has already given us sufficient grace to dis-

cover all of what we are looking for in the midst of our own circumstances.²

5. *Grace is received through humility.* Remember the lines James quotes? "God opposes the proud/ but gives grace to the humble" (James 4:6b). God sometimes allows Satan to inflict a disease such as cancer on us to check the self-centered ego that may be gripping our hearts. Suffering breaks the back of ego and brings us to our knees. Sufficient grace was designed by God to humble Paul. Paul prayed in faith on three occasions that God would heal him. Even for such a one as he, prayers offered in faith are not always answered the way we believe is best.

When we pray with faith for the removal of a disease such as cancer, our sovereign Lord often withholds His healing power. Instead, He gives us the healing power of grace. When we are weak, when we humble ourselves before God, He generates within us endurance to overcome suffering. He replaces pride with humility. Thus we grow through our trials. And that, James says, should bring us joy:

> Consider it pure joy, my brothers, whenever you face trials of many kinds, because you know that the testing of your faith develops perseverance. Perseverance must finish its work so that you may be mature and complete, not lacking anything. (James 1:2–4)

Suffering Christian, What Is it?

Suffering Christian!
What is it that
The harder you work to receive
And the stronger your sense of pride grows
The more you loose its strength?

Suffering Christian!
What is it that
You accept as a gift of unconditional love
And as your weakened pride diminishes
The more you gain its power?

Suffering Christian!
It is God's grace that
He gives to the humble
And His power is made perfect in
  weakness
And through the power of grace you are
  strong!
—John E. Packo

Humbly accepting grace during chemotherapy

I was now scheduled to begin more chemo-therapy—a second series of treatments. Never have I felt so sick, so weak, so helpless for such a long period of time. It was a humbling experience. Just driving to the hospital made me begin to feel nauseated. By now my system had become programmed by the repeated treatments. I knew that I would be vomiting as I returned home. I dreaded the blood tests through the scar tissue that had formed on my veins.

At the hospital I endured the blood drawing and the X-rays. The blood check was necessary to determine whether the counts were at a proper level for more treatments.

Dr. Liepman came briskly down the hall. "OK, John," she said. "You are able to receive the treatment."

"Is it really necessary to continue the chemo, doctor?" I asked. "I am in remission."

"You are not finished with your program yet! You don't want to come back and start all over again, do you? Every cancer cell that the ultrasound machine cannot see must be removed from your system or the multiplication process will rapidly take place again."

"OK." I never questioned Dr. Leipman again.

The new treatments used a different combination of drugs. I received 1,580 milligrams of Cytoxin and 5,900 milligrams of Ara-C to knock out the remaining cancer cells. These drugs made me more violently ill than the first course. This new combination took two and a half hours to drip into my bloodstream. That was longer by far than the first set. After the first hour I became nauseated and began to vomit. The vomiting continued for the rest of the treatment, all the way home and for about six hours after I arrived back home. Those eight hours during each of the final five treatments had to be the most miserable experiences of my entire life.

Returning home from Germany aboard a troop ship in November, 1953, I was seasick. Someone described seasickness as "being too sick to die." That is how I felt during the chemo treatments. But God's grace ministered inner endurance that carried me through those final five treatments.

Chemo increases awareness of suffering

Going through this ordeal time and again increased my awareness of suffering in our world. It came to the point where I could not watch any violence on television. Even a fist fight in a western show would turn my stomach. I became sympathetic toward other cancer patients. I felt the desire to share with as many of them as possible the biblical principles that had helped me cope.

Along with the nausea was the psychological anxiety of anticipating the next treatment. With each succeeding treatment, my anxiety level inched upward a few degrees. I found myself praying again and again, "Oh, Lord, is it really necessary for me to go through all this agony just to live?"

It is ironic that the side effects of these multi-agent anticancer drugs appear to cause more suffering than the disease itself. I have prayed much that a treatment will be discovered soon that obviates the aftereffects of chemotherapy.

The final treatment—finally!

Along with the power of God's grace providing inner endurance for each nausea attack was the knowledge that I had one less treatment to go. I kept count to encourage myself.

The final treatment took place on September 28, 1981. By this time, just the sight of the hospital overwhelmed me with feelings of nausea. The hospital odors added to my misery.

"Remember, John," Elaine reassured me, "this is the last treatment. You won't have to go through this ordeal anymore!"

Since I had experienced so much vomiting in the past, the nurse placed me in a treatment room by myself. I prayed as usual and tried to read to keep my mind off the treatment. But after an hour, the nausea began on schedule. The contents of the bottle appeared to drip at a slower place. The hands of the clock seemed stuck. I had the overwhelming urge to yank the needle from the back of my hand, run from the room and never return! Over and over I repeated Philippians 4:13: "I can do everything through [Christ] who gives me strength."

God's grace gives me endurance, I said to myself. *With God's help I can make it!* And with His help I did! What a sense of relief it was when the technician removed the needle from my hand!

At home, time once again seemed to freeze. I was unusually tired, more so than after the other treatments. About 9:00 p.m. I dozed off, awakening again around 10:30. The nausea had disappeared. What a sense of peace and relief to know that my last bout with nausea was behind me!

As I look back on the six months of treatments I now appreciate more than ever, on a deeper level, the wonder of God's grace. When we humbly allow His grace to work within us, we experience God's unlimited power to carry us through the most difficult places in life. In these hard places we develop a greater dependency on Him. I learned that when God withholds physical healing He gives us the power of His grace to sustain us. It is amazing that through His grace His power increases—as our weakness grows!

Another example of God's grace

Charles W. Colson shares how he prayed for grace during his bout with stomach cancer. The low-grade malignancy had been discovered early. Doctors removed it surgically, giving Colson an excellent prognosis.

As the born-again former White House "hatchet man" was tied to the hospital tubes, he had time to reflect on the larger perspective of God's design in our lives. He said:

If God really delivers His people from all pain and illness, as is so often claimed, why was I so sick? Had my faith become weak? Had I fallen from favor? No. I had always recognized such teaching as false theology. But after four weeks in a maximum-care unit, I came to see it as something else: a presumptuous stumbling block to real evangelism. During my nightly walks through the hospital corridors . . . I often met an Indian man whose two-year-old son had two failed kidney transplants, a brain aneurysm and was now blind for life.

When the father, a Hindu, discovered I was a Christian, he asked if God would heal his son if he, too, was born again. He said he had heard things like that on television. . . .

I told my Hindu friend about Jesus. Yes, He may miraculously intervene in our lives. But we come to God not because of what He may do to spare us suffering, but because Christ is truth. What He does promise us is much more—the forgiveness of sin and eternal life. I left the hospital with my friend studying Christian literature, the Bible and my own account in *Born Again.*[3]

Colson also had this interesting thought to share:

I thought often in the hospital of the words of a Florida pastor. Steve says that every time a nonchristian gets cancer, God allows a Christian to get cancer as well—so the world can see the difference. I prayed I might be so filled with God's grace that the world might see the difference.[4]

Then Colson suggested what he believed was God's purpose for allowing him to experience cancer:

I can only believe that God allowed my cancer for a purpose—just as He allows far more horrific and deadly cancers in fellow Christians every day. We don't begin to know all the reasons why. But we do know that our suffering and weakness can be an opportunity to witness to the world the amazing grace of God at work through us.[5]

Heart-Talk

Emotionally (I feel): I am so bone weary and sick from all the chemo treatments that I feel like giving up. My emotions are experiencing guilt for not having enough faith for a miracle. Then I would not be going through this awful suffering. I would not be feeling as worthless as I do.

Intellectually (I think): I am meditating on the healing Word of God:

> You then, my son, be strong in the grace that is in Christ Jesus. . . . Endure hardship with us like a good soldier of Christ Jesus. (2 Timothy 2:1–3)

> We do not have a high priest who is unable to sympathize with our weaknesses, but we have one who has been tempted in every way, just as we are—yet was without sin. Let us then approach the throne of grace with confidence, so that we may receive mercy and find grace to help us in our time of need. (Hebrews 4:15–16)

[God] gives us more grace. That is why Scripture says:

> "God opposes the proud
>   but gives grace to the humble."
>   (James 4:6)

> The God of all grace, who called you to his eternal glory in Christ, after you have suffered a little while, will himself restore you and make you strong, firm and steadfast. (1 Peter 5:10)

Volitionally (I choose): I will live by grace and not cope with cancer through my own efforts. I humbly choose God's grace to permit His power to be made perfect in my weakness. In my pain I choose to look below the surface of life to develop a greater depth of spirituality and joyful humility.

Prayer

Dear Heavenly Father, I thank You for Your amazing grace. Forgive me for pride that may have kept me from living by grace. I praise You for Calvary love, which shows I am of great value to You. Rid me of feeling guilty that I didn't have enough faith to be healed instantly. I realize that when You withhold healing, You give sufficient grace for every trial. Teach me to accept my suffering with a joyful humility. In Jesus' name, amen.

CREATIVE CHOICE #9:

"I love God who specializes in the miracle of turning cancer into my ultimate spiritual good of Christlikeness."

And we know that in all things God works for the good of those who love him, who have been called according to his purpose. For those God foreknew he also predestined to be conformed to the likeness of his Son.
Romans 8:28–29a

Every trial and difficulty is not an enemy that has come to overwhelm us, but as a divine opportunity to prove something more in the all sufficiency of Christ, and to show something more through which faith can carry us in victory. Then will all earth's mountains become a way, and Satan's stumbling blocks, stones with which to build a stairway to heaven.
A.B. Simpson

Romans 8:28 is the wonder verse that works wonders when bad things happen to good people. For the cancer patient who loves the Lord, it is an incredible promise: "We know that in all things God works for the good of those who love him, who have been called according to his purpose." God promises spiritual good amid all the bad effects of cancer.

As a pastor, I have shared that verse more often than any other with believers who have experienced all types of hardships, including cancer. As a cancer patient myself, I eagerly claimed its promise that I had shared with so many others. It helped me to look at my cancer from God's viewpoint. Turning cancer into spiritual good is a wonder that still amazes me.

Looking at bad events from God's perspective

An excellent analogy that has often been used to describe how bad events fit into God's design is the lesson of the tapestry. Visitors on the main floor, seeing only the back side of the tapestry as it hangs from a high balcony, look at a confusing mass of multicolored threads. They discern no pattern; they are not impressed. But let them climb the stairs to where they can overlook the tapestry in all its splendor, and it becomes for them a breathtaking work of art.

Harold Kushner, in his bestselling book *When Bad Things Happen to Good People,* uses the tapestry illustration and makes this application:

God has a pattern into which all of our lives fit. His pattern requires that some lives be twisted, knotted or cut short, not because one thread is more deserving than another, but simply the pattern requires it. Looked at from underneath, from our vantage point in life, God's pattern of reward and punishment seems arbitrary and without design. But looked at from outside this life, from God's vantage point, every twist and every knot is seen to have its place in a great design.[1]

Romans 8:28 gives us a spiritual view of the knots and twists on the bottom side of the tapestry. They turn out to be the spiritual perfections of Christlikeness on the top side. Let us examine the verse in detail to gain wisdom about God's grand design.

Cancer: God's opportunity to create spiritual good

"In *all things* God works for . . . good." Take that key phrase, "all things," and substitute your own tragedy. If cancer is it, read the verse, "In *cancer* God works for . . . good." Satan is the ultimate cause of creation's "sufferings" (8:18) and "groaning" (8:22), including cancer. Yet God allows suffering, not necessarily because of immoral behavior or bad habits, but to make it possible for us to cooperate with Him for our own spiritual good.

You ask, "Can 'all things' really include cancer?" The context of Romans 8:28 refers to the suffering experienced on earth, including childbirth. This is the particular pain most often mentioned in the Bible. God declares:

> We know that the whole creation has been groaning as in the pains of childbirth right up to the present time. (Romans 8:22)

We are amazed by the miracle of childbirth. That new baby, contentedly asleep between soft white sheets, bears in miniature perfection the physical and mental attributes of parents and even grandparents. But that new life was born out of pain and suffering. If we can let this application grip us, we will realize that pain can be the beginning of a new life of spiritual good.

Suffering in the context of Romans 8:28 includes all the worst circumstances: persecution, tragedy, physical and emotional pain, serious diseases such as cancer. Cancer can cause psychological hurt, physical damage, social rejection and even death. But God can take this tangled mass of heartache and miraculously create from it something spiritually good and beautiful. When we recognize this wonder in His design, we can cooperate with God by coping with cancer in a positive and creative manner.

Building Christlike character for spiritual good

It is essential that we carefully define the word *good*—"We know that in all things God works for the *good* of those who love him." Does *good* refer to material success, prosperity, happiness? Today those things are emphasized. In the case of Job, God restored his wealth twofold, but the greatest, most lasting good was in the area of the patriarch's spiritual life.

The *good* referred to in Romans 8:28 is clearly identified in verse 29a: "For those God foreknew he also predestined to be conformed to the likeness of his Son." God wants to transform our moral natures into Christlikeness. As we cope with cancer, God wants us to realize that He designs to use this sickness to develop moral perfection. Ultimate moral perfection can only be realized as we reach heaven and become like Jesus when we see Him as He is:

> Dear friends, now we are children of God, and what we will be has not yet been made known. But we know that when he appears, we shall be like him, for we shall see him as he is. Everyone who has this hope in him purifies himself, just as he is pure. (1 John 3:2–3)

Whether you are a cancer patient or want to

help such a person to have hope, you may find encouragement from this application. God desires to take our spiritual life and build it into a pillar of moral strength and Christlike character. Instead of becoming a burden too heavy to bear, cancer can become a bridge to lead us into Christlikeness.

A biologist tells how he watched an ant carrying a piece of straw, which seemed a large burden for the creature. The ant came to a crack in the earth too wide for it to cross. It stood for a time as though pondering the situation, then put the straw across the crack and walked across on it![2]

That is a lesson for the cancer patient. Your burden of cancer can be a bridge to lead you into the highest spiritual good of Christlike character.

To create spiritual good, we must love God

"We know that in all things God works for the good of *those who love him.*" This working for good is available to every believer who loves God. All things do not work together for good for everyone. Self-centered people do not naturally love God until the miraculous spiritual birth occurs in their lives. This makes the loving relationship possible. The great motivation behind our spiritual birth was God's love for us. He sent His Son into this sinful, suffering world that we might live through Him:

> This is how God showed his love among us: He sent his one and only Son into the world that we might live through him. This is love: not that we loved God, but that he loved us and sent his Son as an atoning sacrifice for our sins. (1 John 4:9–10)

Love, the highest quality of Christlike character

God's action in Christ has forever changed our understanding of love. Love (*agapao*) is an act of the will in which we give ourselves to God as Christ gave Himself for us on the cross.

Jesus Christ mirrored the love of God in His life and teaching. He emphasized the Old Testament teaching of the law and prophets, which summed up the first and greatest commandment:

> "Love the Lord your God with all your heart and with all your soul and with all your mind." This is the first and greatest commandment. And the second is like it: "Love your neighbor as yourself." (Matthew 22:37–39)

The command to love is so basic that in the great love chapter—First Corinthians 13—we

are warned that even faith cannot substitute:
"If I have a faith that can move mountains, but
have not love, I am nothing" (13:2b). Thus, action that is not motivated by love is nothing in
God's sight. If love moves us to action, we can
be sure we are under the control of the Holy
Spirit and not ourselves. The following diagram
illustrates God's love motivated by His Holy
Spirit within the Christian.

Fruit of the Spirit *Galatians 5:22–23*	*God's love in action* *1 Corinthians 13:1–7*
LOVE	Love never fails. (13:8)
JOY	Love . . . rejoices with the truth. (13:6)
PEACE	Love . . . keeps no record of wrongs. (13:4–5)
PATIENCE	Love is patient. (13:4)
KINDNESS	Love is kind. . . . It is not self-seeking. (13:4–5)
GOODNESS	Love . . . does not envy, . . . does not delight in evil. (13:4–6)
FAITHFULNESS	Love . . . always protects, always trusts, always hopes, always perseveres. (13:6–7)
GENTLENESS	Love . . . does not boast, it is not proud. It is not rude. (13:4–5)
SELF-CONTROL	Love . . . is not easily angered. (13:4–5)

Jesus said, "Whoever has my commands and obeys them, he is the one who loves me" (John 14:21a). And again, "If anyone loves me, he will obey my teaching" (14:23a). The Scriptures say, "This is love for God: to obey his commands" (1 John 5:3a). We evidence our love for God when we give ourselves and all our frailties, including cancer, in complete submission and obedience to God. Our love for God prompts obedience, and this in turn deepens our relationship with God, enabling Him to reveal even more of Himself to us.

Sometimes God finds it necessary to discipline us in order to deepen our relationship with Him. This corrective action is for our spiritual good and proves His love for us. See what the Bible says:

> My son, do not make light of the Lord's
>   discipline,
>   and do not lose heart when he rebukes
>   you,
> because the Lord disciplines those he
>   loves,
>   and he punishes everyone he accepts as a
>   son. (Hebrews 12:5b–6)

This divine discipline brings us into line with the will of God. God's will then becomes our will. His present will to develop Christlikeness in us becomes our will. Our deepening love for God creates in us a desire to realize His spiritual good for us, even though the route is difficult. Once we understand the value of discipline, we will say with the psalmist:

> It was good for me to be afflicted
> so that I might learn your decrees.
> (Psalm 119:71)

In his book *Don't Waste Your Sorrows,* Paul E. Billheimer has this insight for the suffering Christian:

> In the universal absolute sense, there is no character without suffering. Suffering love is the cornerstone of the universe because without it there is no decentralization of the self and therefore no agape love. One who has never voluntarily suffered is totally selfish. Only great sufferers are truly benevolent. There is no such thing as a saint who has not suffered.[3]

Meaning behind suffering reduces stress

It is a well documented fact that a person can much more easily bear up under suffering if he or she can find meaning in it. Seeing suffering from God's viewpoint brings meaning, hope and encouragement. When we come to the place where we see cancer as a means of receiving spiritual good, we can better cope with the stresses it forces upon us. As we look at the underside of the tapestry, we may not be able to understand the twisted threads labeled "cancer." But knowing the Master Craftsman chose to weave them into His pattern of Christlikeness reduces the inevitable stresses. An unknown writer said,

> Behind my life the Weaver stands,
>   And works His wondrous will.
> I leave it in His all-wise hands,
>   And trust His perfect skill;
> Should mystery enshroud His plan,
>   And my short sight be dim,
> I will not try the whole to scan,
>   But leave each thread with Him.
>
> Nor till the loom is silent,
>   And the shuttles cease to fly,
> Shall God unfold the pattern,
>   And explain the reason why
> The dark threads were as needful
>   (In the Master's skillful hand)
> As the threads of gold and silver
>   In the pattern which He planned.

God is able to work for our physical good

God in His sovereignty at times miraculously heals people to cut short their suffering. He has even been known to use mud:

The Pharisees also asked [the former blind man] how he had received his sight. "He put mud on my eyes," the man replied, "and I washed, and now I see." (John 9:15)

I believe God can use the medical profession to bring physical healing. Our challenge is to love God and grow in Christlikeness, whether God intervenes directly or uses doctors in the healing process.

On October 20, 1981, seven months after the diagnosis of lymphoma, Elaine and I had an appointment with Dr. Miller to receive an evaluation. He greeted us with a reassuring smile.

"This morning," he began, "a group of us doctors had a conference. We looked over your file. We all came to one conclusion: You are a miracle!" Elaine and I were overjoyed.

"We are grateful for this miracle," my wife said to Dr. Miller. "We thank the Lord for His healing power." The two of us left the hospital deeply grateful for extended life and for God's still-intact promise to bless the latter years more than the first.

The Lord is faithful to His promises. I received word that my manuscript, *Find and Use Your Spiritual Gifts,* based on my doctoral dissertation, was being published. A number of new families had become a part of our congregation, nearly doubling its size. Someone asked me how I accounted for the sudden numerical surge in our church's size. "Chemo," I answered, tongue-in-cheek. Then, on a serious note, I added, "It was entirely of the Lord, for I was unable to visit them. It is a fulfillment of the Lord's promise to grant me a greater ministry. We have seen the beginning of that promise."

Heart-Talk

Emotionally (I feel): I feel God has turned His back on me and that life is unfair. I am perplexed. Did I do something terrible to suffer like this?

Intellectually (I think): I am meditating on the healing Word of God:

> We also rejoice in our sufferings, because we know that suffering produces perseverance; perseverance, character, and character, hope. And hope does not disappoint us, because God has poured out his love into our hearts by the Holy Spirit, whom he has given us. (Romans 5:3–5)

> Dear friends, now we are children of God, and what we will be has not yet been made known. But we know that when he appears, we shall be like him, for we shall see him as he is. (1 John 3:2)

> My son, do not make light of the Lord's
>   discipline,
>   and do not lose heart when he rebukes
>   you,
> because the Lord disciplines those he
>   loves,
>   and he punishes everyone he accepts as a
>   son. (Hebrews 12:5b–6)

Volitionally (I choose): I choose to love God with all my heart, mind and strength. I will not lose heart when God disciplines me, for this is the proof of the Father's love for me. I will rejoice in suffering, which will lead to a Christlike character.

Prayer

Dear loving Heavenly Father, I worship You for Your unfailing love. You are disciplining me to be more like Jesus. May my love for You grow greatly. Help me to focus on Jesus, who suffered for me. Forgive me for complaining of my aches and pains. I rejoice that when Jesus appears, I shall be like Him. In Jesus' name, amen.

"I dedicate my body to Christ and separate it from unhealthy eating habits, chemical abuse and overexposure to sun."

Don't you know that you yourselves are God's temple and that God's Spirit lives in you? If anyone destroys God's temple, God will destroy him: for God's temple is sacred, and you are that temple.
1 Corinthians 3:16–17

Men go abroad to wonder at the height of the mountains, at the huge waves of the sea, at the long courses of the rivers, at the vast compass of the ocean, at the circular motion of the stars, and they pass by themselves without wondering. Saint Augustine

Studies show that former cancer patients live healthier lives than before the disease struck. Too many of us take our bodies for granted. Augustine referred to this frame of mind when he observed that people "pass by themselves without wondering." But those of us who have or have had cancer know that we are wonderfully put together. We no longer take life for granted. With the psalmist we can sing:

> I praise you because I am fearfully and
> wonderfully made;
> your works are wonderful,
> I know that full well. (Psalm 139:14)

God marvelously designed our bodies to grow, to act and react, to rule their own activities and to repair themselves. He also gave these bodies the ability to reproduce themselves, assuring the continuity of life. In view of God's amazingly creative handiwork, we have a responsibility to properly care for our bodies.

As a former cancer patient, I have not only a greater-than-ever respect for my body but a new zeal to care for it in hopes of keeping it cancer-free. I am careful to practice "preventive healing" stressed by the medical profession. I get timely cooperation from my oncologist, who sees that I receive pamphlets explaining the importance of healthy diets and activities and who updates me on the latest medical findings.

Preventive healing has priority

Preventive healing actually had its beginning in the early history of Israel. As the nation left

Egypt enroute to the land of promise, God set forth preventive measures to guard the health of His people. Observing these regulations was part of an Israelite's spiritual loyalty. As Robert G. Witty observes, these health and dietary measures had priority over restorative healing:

> Before God revealed that "I am the God that healeth thee," He first promised that "I will put none of these diseases upon thee" (Exodus 15:26). From the first, God rated healing as second best to health. Preventive healing by obedience preceded restorative healing.[1]

There is a growing awareness among the medical profession that observing these biblical principles is effective in the prevention of many diseases. S.I. McMillen, M.D., in his book *None of These Diseases*, writes:

> Medical science is still discovering how obedience to the ancient prescriptions saved the primitive Hebrews from the scourges of epidemic plagues; and medical research is constantly proving the timeless potency of the divine prescriptions for modern diseases.[2]

Two examples of preventive healing

Dr. McMillen cites two examples to show that the biblical principles are timeless.

1. Obedience to the ancient law of separating those with leprosy from the general public erased that disease in Europe. When the leprosy epidemic of the Dark Ages raged out of control and the physicians had nothing to offer, the church pressed for the isolation of the leprous "outside the camp" as described in Leviticus 13:46. As a result, leprosy was checked and eventually eliminated.[3]

2. God decreed sanitary rules for the disposal of human waste (Deuteronomy 23:12–13). Poor sanitary habits in Europe up until the end of the 18th century brought widespread death from diseases like typhoid, cholera and dysentery. Most of those deaths could have been prevented had people taken seriously God's ancient ordinance.[4]

Cancer prevention is as vital as its cure

In 1984 the National Cancer Institute conducted a nationwide survey. They discovered that "half of Americans think 'everything causes cancer' and there is not much a person can do to prevent cancer." According to the Institute, this misinformed attitude is actually contributing indirectly to nearly 100,000 cancer deaths each year. The Institute oversees the federal government's billion-dollar-a-year battle against cancer. Of the billion dollars, the Institute has earmarked one million dollars for a program to make cancer prevention a national reality. Contrary to widespread opinion, "everything" does not cause cancer.[5]

My doctor's advice for preventing a recurrence

After Dr. Miller announced my "miracle" recovery from cancer, he instructed me about preventive measures I could take to reduce chances of its return. He prescribed no medication. Rather, he encouraged me to follow these rules to preserve the good health that had returned to my body:

1. Eat proper foods.
2. Abstain from cigarette smoking.
3. Keep body weight normal for age and height.
4. Keep emotional stresses at the lowest possible levels.
5. Have a yearly physical examination.

It was not until I began to read and clip articles about cancer that I began to understand how a few simple preventive measures could have such amazing results.

Reducing the risk of cancer

The best news about cancer and a major topic of discussion in the medical profession is cancer prevention. Scientists have discovered many factors that contribute to cancer. They estimate that 80 percent of all cancers may be related to the environment and the things we eat, drink and breathe. The remaining 20 percent can be attributed to things we cannot control, such as a family predisposition to cancer. If, therefore, we change the things we can control, we can greatly reduce our risk of cancer. The figures in the diagram below, compiled by the National Cancer Institute, show the leading causes of death by cancer.

Diet	35%
Tobacco	30%
Infection	10%
Reproductive and Sexual Behavior	7%
Occupation	4%
Pollution	2%
Others	5%

A holy body: God's "preventive healing"

The Bible stresses the sanctity of the body and makes us responsible for its proper care. The body is sacred for three biblical reasons:

1. God created the body as the present and eternal home of our spirit and soul. The human body also became the eternal form of the incarnate Christ Himself. Albert B. Simpson makes this observation:

The reason why God has so honored the

human form is very clear in the subsequent revelation of Jesus Christ and the great mystery of the incarnation. It was because the human body was designed to be the ultimate climax of the whole creation and the eternal form of the incarnate God Himself. Always, it would seem, the Lord Jesus Christ had purposed to become embodied in a human form and to link the creation with the Creator in His own wonderful Person.[6]

2. The body is sacred because the Holy Spirit indwells the believer. Paul made this clear to the Corinthian Christians:

Don't you know that you yourselves are God's temple and that God's Spirit lives in you? If anyone destroys God's temple, God will destroy him; for God's temple is sacred, and you are that temple. (1 Corinthians 3:16–17)

3. God owns us and therefore, as stewards, we are responsible to care for these bodies that belong to Him:

You are not your own; you were bought at a price. Therefore honor God with your body. (1 Corinthians 6:19b–20)

Two aspects of the word *sanctify* must be considered in the stewardship of body, soul and spirit. First, *sanctify* means to separate. We have the responsibility to separate our bodies from all known harmful effects.

> Come out from them
>   and be separate,
>   says the Lord.
> Touch no unclean thing,
>   and I will receive you.
>   (2 Corinthians 6:17)

When we recognize that certain foods and other substances such as tobacco and alcohol are leading causes of cancer, we should voluntarily separate ourselves—meaning our bodies—from them.

Second, *sanctify* means to dedicate. To dedicate is to separate to. We are not only to separate our bodies from harmful substances and activities, but as we recognize God's ownership of our bodies we are to replace the harmful with what is healthy. Eating what is good for us pleases God because it demonstrates to Him that we want to care for our bodies—His temples. We should be asking ourselves whether our eating habits glorify and honor the Lord Jesus Christ and His Holy Spirit.

Sanctification's two-way action

Paul has some pertinent comments in Ephesians 4:22–32, demonstrating the two-way action of "separating from" and "separating to." He speaks of "putting off" and "putting on." When we attempt to separate ourselves from something unhealthy, it needs to be as good as dead if we are going to experience deliverance from it. Note in the following diagram what we are to "put off" and what we are to "put on."

Putting Sanctification into Action

"Put off" Separate from:	"Put on" Dedicate to:
Old self (v. 22)	New self (v. 23)
Falsehood (v. 25)	Speak truth (v. 25)
Stealing (v. 28)	Do useful work (v. 28)
Unwholesome talk (v. 29)	Edifying talk (v. 29)
Bitterness, rage, anger, brawling, slander, malice (v. 31)	Kindness, compassion, forgiveness (v. 31)

Are we not to follow the same actions of "putting off" and "putting on" for the health of the body as we are instructed to do for the health of the soul and spirit? In "putting off," we separate ourselves from unhealthy substances and activities that are leading causes of cancer; in "putting on," we dedicate ourselves to eating healthy food and participating in healthy activities. We are creative when we practice sanctification God's way. God is able to give us bodies with healthy immune systems, healthy lungs, healthy digestive systems. It is our responsibility to chose to practice sanctification for the whole person, and God follows our commitment with His enabling power. We separate ourselves, and God makes the separation good.

Those of us who are believers have a tremendous advantage over nonbelievers in the prevention of cancer. God not only asks us to keep from unhealthy practices and replace them with healthful ones, but the Holy Spirit within us is faithful to give us His power to do so. The apostle Paul offered this prayer:

> May God himself, the God of peace, sanctify you through and through. May your whole spirit, soul and body be kept blameless at the coming of our Lord Jesus Christ. The one who calls you is faithful and he will do it. (1 Thessalonians 5:23–24)

Dedicated to a healthy diet

If the leading cause of all cancer (35 percent) is related to what we eat, is it not reasonable to become knowledgeable about healthy foods?

Should we not choose to practice sanctification for preventive healing of the digestive system?

The Bible nowhere proscribes meat as food, and, indeed, by implication approves it for the human diet. Nevertheless, Daniel, the prophet-statesman of Israel's exile, somewhat inadvertently became the father of today's high fiber diet. During his three-year training program in Babylon, the king order that Daniel eat the royal food and drink the king's wine. Rather than eat food and drink wine that had been offered first to heathen gods, Daniel and his three Jewish associates, Hananiah, Mishael and Azariah, proposed a much different diet and a 10-day test:

> "Give us nothing but vegetables to eat and water to drink. Then compare our appearance with that of the young men who eat the royal food." . . . At the end of the ten days they looked healthier and better nourished than any of the young men who ate the royal food. (Daniel 1:12b–15)

The Hebrew word for *vegetables* used here implies leguminous plants such as lentils, peas and beans. In asking for these vegetables, Daniel and his friends were requesting a diet high in fiber. Ten days later, all four who ate the high fiber diet "looked healthier and better nourished" than those who ate the king's diet.[7]

Fiber: a vital ingredient for a healthy diet

Bill Gothard, well-known Christian lecturer, presented a fascinating paper to the 1986 All-Day Minister's Seminar he held in leading cities across the United States. Its title: "How the Analogy of Christ to Bread Gives Direction for Avoiding Diseases." Gothard wrote:

> By studying the life and ministry of Christ and the newest medical research on the preparation and use of bread, we are able to discover significant correlations between them. . . . Applying them to our preparation and consumption of bread will be the avoidance of many common diseases in our day.[8]

When Jesus said, "I am the bread of life," He was drawing a spiritual analogy. He is the main staple of spiritual life just as fibrous wheat bread was once the main staple of physical life. Wheat bread has continued to be the major staple in many third-world countries. Where this is the case, an amazing number of diseases experienced in Western civilization are not found.

Gothard's primary medical research for his paper was provided by Denis Burkitt, M.D., of London, formerly a missionary doctor in Africa. Burkitt won world acclaim for his major role in uncovering the causes and pioneering the cure for a form of cancer in children. He is also noted as a key figure in confirming the link between many serious diseases of the Western world and the lack of fiber in our diets.

In countries where appendicitis, diverticular disease, hiatus hernia, hemorrhoids, coronary disease and colon-rectal cancer are rare, high fiber bread is a major staple of the diet. The common denominator of all these diseases is a lack of fiber, which, in turn, causes constipation. Dr. Burkitt calls the United States "a constipated nation from the Atlantic coast to the Pacific."[9] He relates the low incidence of Western diseases in other countries to a more rapid transit of the food residue in the digestive tract. This is made possible through more fiber intake. Dr. Burkitt reaches this conclusion:

> Your chance of a long healthy life is more directly related to the amount of stool you pass daily than to your blood pressure, your glucose tolerance curves, your serum cholesterol and many other things the doctor examines when you see him.[10]

Studies published in the *Journal of the National Cancer Institute* show evidence that dietary fiber can reduce the risk of colon-rectal cancer. Each year that disease strikes more than 150,000 Americans, and kills more than 60,000.

It was reported in *The New York Times* that fiber can shrink some polyps:

> The findings are the first to show in people that an ordinary food, in this case a cereal rich in bran, can reverse the usual progression to cancer. . . . Dr. Peter Greenwald of the National Cancer Institute said this was especially important for people with a family history of colon-rectal cancer, who are three times more likely than the average American to develop it themselves.[11]

The diets of the ancient Israelites included both grains and fruit. Before the Israelites entered Canaan, the region was described as "a land with wheat and barley, vines and fig trees, pomegranates, olive oil and honey; a land where bread will not be scarce" (Deuteronomy 8:8–9a). Since the people of that day did not refine their flour as we do today, their bread was made from whole grains that were rich in fiber. Furthermore, they did not eat large amounts of unsaturated fats. Most animals were pasture-fed and their fat was not eaten. They used olive oil for cooking. Instead of refined sugar, they used honey.

Dedicating the body to clean lungs

Lung cancer accounts for 30 percent of all cancer deaths. This disease was rare in the

early 1900s, but today it is claiming over
100,000 lives a year in the United States alone.
Lung cancer was once primarily a male disease.
Today, with a record number of women smoking, it is the leading cause of cancer deaths
among women, surpassing even breast cancer.

What is the answer? Sanctification. By
separating the body from cigarette smoking,
the major cause of lung cancer, the chances of
getting this type of cancer can be greatly
reduced.

Once as I was doing some pastoral visiting, I
met a man in his mid 20s who pulled up his
sport shirt to show me patches of darkened
skin. He said he had had radium treatments.
As he spoke, he was dragging on a cigarette.

"I believe God is going to heal me so completely of cancer," he bragged, "that even my
skin color will come back to normal." Six weeks
later he was dead. Had he separated himself
from smoking, he might have avoided an early
death. It is remarkable to me how many people
I meet in the waiting rooms of hospitals who
still smoke although they are there for treatment of lung cancer. It is estimated that in an
18-hour waking day:

> . . . a two-pack-a-day smoker spends from
> three to four hours with a cigarette in
> mouth, hand or ash tray, takes about 400
> puffs for the day and inhales up to 1,000
> milligrams of tar. . . . [Such a person has]

three times the risk of death from heart attack and nearly twenty times the risk of death from lung cancer [as the non-smoker].[12]

Separating the body from alcohol

The heavy user of alcoholic beverages, especially in combination with smoking, can cause cancer of the liver, esophagus, mouth and larynx. The use of alcohol has also been suspect in breast cancer. John Noble, of *The New York Times*, reported that new studies conclude women appear to place themselves at a higher risk of developing breast cancer if they take as few as three alcoholic drinks a week:

> The findings, published . . . in *The New England Journal of Medicine*, provide the strongest evidence yet of an apparent link between drinking and breast cancer. They supported several earlier findings that indicated an association and went further in suggesting that even relatively light drinking could be dangerous.[13]

Separating the body from sun worship

Despite repeated warnings from the American Cancer Society, every summer sees our beaches crowded with sun bathers. It is estimated that most of the 400,000 cases of non-melanoma skin cancer contracted each year in the United States are sun-related. Studies show that the major cause of the deadly melanoma is overexposure to the sun's ultraviolet rays. With the enlarging hole in the layer of ozone that protects us from ultraviolet rays, researchers expect this sun-related cancer to increase. Preventive measures for those who must be in the sun are relatively simple: sunscreens, broad-brimmed hats, clothing that covers otherwise exposed skin surfaces.

Our human bodies are the only ones we will have in this lifetime. They have been given to us by God as instruments of His righteousness. Let us not permit secular thinking to mold us in its unsanctified lifestyles. It is reasonable for us to submit our bodies to God as a spiritual act of worship. After all, our bodies belong to Him; He made them!

> I urge you, brothers, in view of God's mercy, to offer your bodies as living sacrifices, holy and pleasing to God—this is your spiritual act of worship. Do not conform any longer to the pattern of the world, but be transformed by the renewing of your mind. Then you will be able to test and approve what God's will is—his good, pleasing and perfect will. (Romans 12:1–2)

Heart-Talk

Emotionally (I feel): Although I have kept my

body from cancer-causing substances such as tobacco and alcohol, I feel guilty about my unwholesome eating habits. When I get upset I feed my face. I enjoy fried pork chops, french fries, white bread and a large piece of pie a la mode for dessert. And then there are the between-meal snacks of donuts during coffee breaks and chocolate candy, salty chips, peanuts and pretzels, washed down by Cokes, in the evenings. I feel guilty that I have abused my body and have lowered myself to become a glutton, a chocoholic and a junk food junkie.

Intellectually (I think): I will meditate on these healing verses to help me overcome my emotional crutch of food:

> Do not be wise in your own eyes;
>   fear the Lord and shun evil.
> This will bring health to your body
>   and nourishment to your bones.
>   (Proverbs 3:7–8)

> Do not join those who drink too much
>   wine
>   or gorge themselves on meat,
> for drunkards and gluttons become poor,
>   and drowsiness clothes them in rags.
>   (Proverbs 23:20–21)

> Don't you know that you yourselves are God's temple and that God's Spirit lives in

you? If anyone destroys God's temple, God will destroy him; for God's temple is sacred, and you are that temple. (1 Corinthians 3:16–17)

I urge you, brothers, in view of God's mercy, to offer your bodies as living sacrifices, holy and pleasing to God—this is your spiritual act of worship. (Romans 12:1)

Volitionally (I choose): I choose to separate my body, through the inner power of the Holy Spirit, from the known causes of cancer that I can control. I dedicate my body to God, who will be pleased when I maintain a healthy diet. This will include fiber from fresh fruits, vegetables and whole grains along with low-fat meats such as chicken, turkey and fish in moderate portions. I will continue to abstain from smoking and alcohol. And I will exercise.

Prayer
Dear Heavenly Father, I bow in awe at the infinite wisdom You demonstrated when You created our human bodies. You further honored our bodies by sending us Your Son enfleshed in one of them. Then You raised Him from the dead with a glorified body that will exist eternally. I praise You that my body is indwelt by Your Holy Spirit and therefore sacred. Fill me with Your Spirit. Enable me to

separate my body from an unhealthy diet and from other substances that will harm it. Forgive me for judging others' sins when I myself have been mastered by food. I dedicate my body to You. It is my act of spiritual worship and the only reasonable thing to do. In Jesus' name, amen.

"I accept death as the departure into heaven made possible by the resurrection of Jesus Christ from the dead."

Jesus said to her, "I am the resurrection and the life. He who believes in me will live, even though he dies; and whoever lives and believes in me will never die.
John 11:25–26a

There is one great fact which gives the Christian assurance in the face of death: the resurrection of Jesus Christ. It is the physical, bodily resurrection of Christ that gives us confidence and hope. Because Christ rose from the dead, we know beyond doubt that death is not the end, but it is merely the transition to eternal life.[1] Billy Graham

Death is a fact of life that must be faced sooner or later. All of us know it will come, but we do not like to think about dying. We think of it as happening to others, but somehow we act as though we are indestructible. The United States Department of Health and Human Services recognizes death as one of the four greatest fears a patient has when given a diagnosis of cancer. If the cancer is judged to be terminal, the patient must face and cope with the personal reality of death.

People have tried to put life and death in perspective for the cancer patient. Ann Landers wrote, "Life is terminal, cancer isn't."[2] A patient with advanced cancer expressed his view about dying this way: "The death rate for any generation is 100 percent. We all die. However, I know what probably will kill me, and most people don't."

Coupled with the fear of death is anxiety about the suffering that precedes death. The whole painful process leading up to that last gasp for breath is sometimes feared more than death itself. We are afraid that we will not be able to tolerate those conditions. We want to die gracefully.

I know from personal experience the process of sorting through the reality of death and especially the suffering preceding death. I was not given much hope by the doctors. The diagnosis of diffuse histiocytic lymphoma in the advanced stage with approximately one month to live left little room for negotiation. Thankfully, I was prepared to die, if that was the will of God for me.

As a pastor, I had preached to and counseled

people about facing death. One of the rewarding experiences of being a pastor is to minister to those who are on their deathbeds. What a joy to share with them the hope of heaven made possible through Christ's death and resurrection. I have seen many Christians who were at peace with God in their closing moments in this life. They radiated bold faith, remarkable courage and complete trust in God. They were an inspiration to my own faith. I reasoned that if they were able to tolerate the dying process so gracefully, certainly God would also carry me through death and on to heaven. I knew the answer to their courage would be mine as well when the time came.

There is no greater creative choice in the face of possible death than to fill our thinking with the miracle of the resurrection. Keeping our hearts focused on this wonder drives away the fear of death. Fear is replaced with the joyful anticipation of being caught up to an eternal existence with God.

The resurrection of Jesus is a fact

The resurrection of Jesus Christ from the dead is a historic fact which proves that there is life after death. This gives the cancer patient who is a Christian courage and hope in the face of death. The Bible sets forth this great historic event very clearly:

For what I received I passed on to you as

of first importance: that Christ died for our sins according to the Scriptures, that he was buried, that he was raised on the third day according to the Scriptures. (1 Corinthians 15:3–4)

The resurrection is believed to be the greatest miracle in recorded history. It is the one miracle upon which the foundation of Christianity stands. The cross of Christ without the resurrection is meaningless. The resurrection proved God's acceptance of Christ's atoning sacrifice, which is the core of the Christian faith. Christianity stands or falls on the miracle of the resurrection of Christ.

Many brilliant men throughout history have examined in detail the accounts of Christ's death and resurrection more than any other recorded event in history. They have accepted the resurrection as a proven fact. One such skeptic was Frank Morrison, a British lawyer whose goal was to write a book discrediting the resurrection. After he carefully studied the evidence, however, he had a dramatic change of mind and became a believer himself. He wrote a book entitled *Who Moved the Stone?*, which sets forth the evidences for the resurrection of Christ.

Luke the physician wrote this summary of the convincing proofs of the resurrection:

After [Jesus'] suffering, he showed himself

to these men and gave many convincing proofs that he was alive. He appeared to them over a period of forty days and spoke about the kingdom of God. (Acts 1:3)

Looking at mud or the stars?

The cancer patient can have hope in the historic fact that Jesus Christ was resurrected from the dead. This takes away the fear of death, for the resurrection proves that an afterlife exists. Frederick Langbridge poetically relates how two people react to the same distressing situation:

> Two men look out through the same bars;
> One sees mud, and one the stars.[3]

Those who look to medical science and technology alone are looking at mud as far as death is concerned. The Christian, on the other hand, recognizes the limitations of medicine and looks up to the ultimate miracle of the resurrection for courage and hope. He or she looks at the stars. Jesus declared:

> I am the resurrection and the life. He who believes in me will live, even though he dies; and whoever lives and believes in me will never die. (John 11:25–26a)

What happens at physical death?

When I conduct a funeral for a believer, I remind the listeners that the body of their loved one is all that remains in the casket. The soul/spirit has departed from the body to be present with Jesus. Jesus said to the dying thief, after his confession of faith: "I tell you the truth, today you will be with me in paradise" (Luke 23:43). Paul talked of his "earthly tent"—his body—being destroyed and then of his becoming clothed with "an eternal house in heaven, not built by human hands" (2 Corinthians 5:1). About this he adds, "We are confident, I say, and would prefer to be away from the body and at home with the Lord" (5:8).

Clearly, the believer's spirit, which is eternal, will live in the presence of Jesus forever. Death is not to be feared by Christians, for God is with them before, during and after the death experience:

> Even though I walk
>   through the valley of the shadow of
>   death,
> I will fear no evil,
>   . for you are with me;
> your rod and your staff,
>   they comfort me. (Psalm 23:4)

For the Christian, six comforting figures

The Bible, in its inspired imagery, presents six figures of death for the Christian. Each is calculated to inspire confidence for the one walking through "the valley of the shadow of death."

1. *Death is the Christian's coronation.* Death is the end of conflict and the beginning of glory in heaven. The elderly Paul says to his young protege, Timothy:

> Now there is in store for me the crown of righteousness, which the Lord, the righteous Judge, will award to me on that day—and not only to me, but also to all who have longed for his appearing. (2 Timothy 4:8)

2. *Death is a rest from labor.* John the apostle heard a "voice from heaven" saying,

> "Write: Blessed are the dead who die in the Lord from now on."
> "Yes," says the Spirit, "they will rest from their labor, for their deeds will follow them." (Revelation 14:13)

3. *Death marks the beginning, not the end, of a journey.* Paul announced with a note of triumph, "The time has come for my departure"

(2 Timothy 4:6b). The word *departure* literally means "to pull up anchor and to set sail." Thus, death is the beginning, not the end, of a journey.

4. *Death is a transition.* In a text we already looked at, Paul says, "We know that if the earthly tent we live in is destroyed, we have a building from God, an eternal house in heaven, not built by human hands" (2 Corinthians 5:1). To the Christian, death is exchanging a temporary tent for an eternal house. At death we forsake this crumbling, spent body and move into an everlasting dwelling not made with hands.

5. *Death is an exodus.* We speak of being deceased as though it were the end of everything. But the word *deceased* literally means "exodus" or "going out." The imagery is that of the children of Israel triumphantly leaving Egypt and their former life of slavery for the promised land, Canaan.

6. *Death ushers us into a prepared place.* God has provided for all believers a place He calls "many rooms" or resting places (John 14:1–6). When believers die, there is a place in heaven already prepared for them. They will spend eternity with God.

Future miracle: the resurrection of the body

The Scriptures describe a future resurrection

of our human bodies that staggers our imaginations!

> Listen, I tell you a mystery: We will not all sleep, but we will all be changed—in a flash, in the twinkling of an eye, at the last trumpet. For the trumpet will sound, the dead will be raised imperishable, and we will be changed. (1 Corinthians 15:51–52)

The resurrection of our human bodies is a part of the final process in God's plan that leads ultimately to the complete elimination of death. Death is the last enemy to be destroyed (1 Corinthians 15:26). This miraculous change will occur in a split second of time, eliminating any possibility of an evolutionary process.

The key word is *changed*—"we will all be changed." *Changed* is the English translation of the Greek word *metamorphow*, from which we get our word *metamorphosis*. We use the term to describe the tremendous change that takes place when an earthbound caterpillar becomes a free butterfly. The caterpillar spins itself into a tomb. When spring comes, this dead and formless mass emerges as a beautiful butterfly that flutters into the sunny sky.

Cancer can result in disfigurement and ugly scars. But to the believer, this is a temporary condition. Paul might have been expressing the hope of the Christian suffering from terminal cancer when he said,

Our citizenship is in heaven. And we eagerly await a Savior from there, the Lord Jesus Christ, who, by the power that enables him to bring everything under his control, will transform our lowly bodies so that they will be like his glorious body. (Philippians 3:20–21)

Our "lowly bodies" will be transformed into glorified, perfect and eternal bodies that will never again be subject to any form of disease or death. They will be like the glorified body of Jesus. The Scriptures say so: "We know that when [Jesus] appears, we shall be like him, for we shall see him as he is" (1 John 3:2b).

Before and after the resurrection

In First Corinthians 15:42–44, Paul makes a detailed comparison between our bodies prior to the resurrection and our bodies after the resurrection. I have charted these comparisons in the following diagram:

Before	*After*
Sown a perishable body, subject to decay.	Raised an imperishable body, no more decay.
Sown in dishonor. Death is life defeated by sin.	Raised in glory. Perfection is adapted to the new glorified earth.
Sown in weakness. Disease and age robs its strength.	Raised in power, enormous strength to serve God without weariness.

| Sown a natural body governed by physical senses, gravity and time. | Raised a spiritual body with spiritual dimensions to enjoy eternal blessings. |

The diagram uses the word *sown*. The apostle Paul used the term in response to two questions asked by the believers in Corinth: "How are the dead raised? With what kind of body will they come?" (1 Corinthians 15:35).

Paul replies to their questions by appealing to their sense of logic. "What you sow does not come to life unless it dies. When you sow, you do not plant the body that will be, but just a seed" (15:36b–37a). Paul was comparing the miracle of the resurrection of the body to the miracle of the seed, sown in soil, that changes into a plant.

Can you remember your first experience of landscaping your home? You may have sent for a seed catalog with photos of beautiful flowers of every variety. You dreamed of choice places to add beauty and color to your landscape; then you mailed your order. Finally the seeds and bulbs arrived carefully packed and marked. Perhaps like me you eyed the dry, dead-looking bulbs and said to yourself, "How will these ugly brown clumps ever change into the soft, silky daffodils I saw in the catalog?" But in faith you carefully followed the instructions, burying the bulbs and seeds at the right depth, adding water as specified. And with predictable timing, the resurrection happened! First, tiny green blades pierced the brown soil. The green blades grew upward; stalks of buds appeared. Eventually, beautiful splashes of color transformed your landscape as flowers opened their delicate petals to the sunshine.

The same Lord who resurrects ugly bulbs into beautiful daffodils, who transforms repulsive caterpillars into beautiful butterflies will at the resurrection produce miraculous changes in our bodies. And there may be something still more wonderful for the Christian.

Some will totally avoid physical death

Did you agree, at the beginning of this chapter, with the cancer patient who said the death rate for any generation is 100 percent? According to the Bible, there is a generation coming whose death rate will not be 100 percent! Not all will die physically. Christians living when Jesus returns to earth will be physically "changed—in a flash, in the twinkling of an eye" (1 Corinthians 15:51–52), without dying. The "perishable" will "clothe itself with the imperishable, and the mortal with immortality" (15:53). And so they and we shall be with the Lord Jesus Christ forever. Comforting thought!

> The Lord himself will come down from heaven, with a loud command, with the voice of the archangel and with the trumpet call of God, and the dead in Christ will rise first. After that, we who are still alive

and are left will be caught up together with them in the clouds to meet the Lord in the air. And so we will be with the Lord forever. Therefore encourage each other with these words. (1 Thessalonians 4:16–18)

Heart-Talk

Emotionally (I feel): I'm afraid of the pain that comes with dying. I fear death and what the future holds. I don't want to die. I can't believe that this is happening to me.

Intellectually (I think): I am meditating on these healing verses:

> Do not be afraid. I am the First and the Last. I am the Living One; I was dead, and behold I am alive for ever and ever! (Revelation 1:17c–18b)

> Jesus said to her, "I am the resurrection and the life. He who believes in me will live, even though he dies; and whoever lives and believes in me will never die." (John 11:25–26a)

> In his great mercy he has given us new birth into a living hope through the resurrection of Jesus Christ from the dead, and into an inheritance that can never perish,

spoil or fade—kept in heaven for you, who through faith are shielded by God's power until the coming of the salvation that is ready to be revealed in the last time. In this you greatly rejoice, though now for a little while you may have had to suffer grief in all kinds of trials. (1 Peter 1:3b–6)

Volitionally (I choose): I choose to let thoughts of the resurrection fill my mind and replace thoughts of the fear of death. I choose to live in the hope that Jesus may return at any moment, and I will be raptured and changed into spiritual, mental and bodily perfection.

Prayer

Dear Heavenly Father, I marvel at the wonder of the resurrection that awaits every believer. I worship You, Lord Jesus, for Your death and resurrection. This gives me the assurance of an afterlife with You and all the family of God. How grateful I am to be serving a living Savior. I eagerly await Your return to transform this body of mine into a glorious body. And if I should die before that day, it will be with the expectation, an instant later, of being in Your presence in heaven! In Jesus' name, amen.

"I celebrate the wonder of life by filling my heart with the joy of worshiping Jesus."

A cheerful hear is good medicine, but a crushed spirit dries up the bones.
Proverbs 17:22

Do not grieve, for the joy of the Lord is your strength. Nehemiah 8:10c

To him who sits on the throne and to the Lamb be praise and honor and glory and power, for ever and ever. Revelation 5:13b

---

Worship is a celebration that puts me in touch with the truth that shapes my whole life, and I have found it to be a necessary element for my own spiritual formation.[1]
Robert Webber

As a result of having had cancer, I have learned three valuable lessons about worship. First, worship is more meaningful when Christ is at the center of my life. Second, worshiping Jesus is the greatest celebration in life. Third, a worshipful attitude brings the healing strength of joy.

I remember it vividly. Two mornings after my final chemotherapy treatment, as I had my morning devotional time with God, my heart was filled with worship. When I stepped outdoors afterward, the sky appeared bluer, the puffy clouds whiter, the fall foliage more colorful, the sun's smile friendlier. I felt like a child in wide-eyed wonder seeing a brightly colored ball for the first time. Perhaps Ronald B. Allen expressed this wonder best when he wrote:

> Let us therefore luxuriate in our humanity. God help us to become childlike (not childish) in developing again our senses of wonder. It was in wonder that we were made, and it is in wonder that we worship God. As we see the good and lovely things that man can do, let us praise God for this wonder. And as we see the mystery and wonder in creation, let us praise God that we can participate in it.[2]

Celebrating Christ together

When do we celebrate our spiritual life with our family and friends? We celebrate it on Sunday in church. Since the birthday of the church on the day of Pentecost, this celebration has taken place every Sunday morning for nearly

2,000 years—marking the day of Christ's resurrection from the dead. At Pentecost 3,000 people were born into the kingdom of God to begin a new life of worship. Filled with the Holy Spirit, they worshiped the Lord together. As a pastor, one of the joys of ministry is leading my congregation in worship. I am carrying on a tradition for which the church exists. A.W. Tozer said:

> Yes, worship of the loving God is man's whole reason for existence. That is why we are born and that is why we are born again from above. That is why we are created and that is why we have been recreated. That is also why there is a church. The Christian church exists to worship God first of all. Everything else must come second or third or fourth or fifth.[3]

Our worship of God centers around the combined events of Christ's birth, His perfect life, His crucifixion, death, burial, resurrection, bodily ascension to heaven and return to earth to set up His eternal kingdom.

The church has many symbols to assist it in the joy of celebration. The Communion is an example. It is a memorial celebrated with thanksgiving to Christ because He paid with His shed blood the price of our redemption and purchased for us a place in heaven.

After Leonardo da Vinci had finished his

masterpiece *The Last Supper*, he invited a friend to inspect it.

The friend was impressed. "The goblet is wonderful," he exclaimed. "It stands out like solid silver."

Instantly da Vinci snatched a brush and with a stroke erased the goblet from the canvas. "Nothing shall draw the eye of the beholder from my Lord!" da Vinci explained to his friend.

Symbols exist in the church not to be adored but as objects to teach us to magnify and worship Jesus Christ. Likewise, we exist not to worship self, but to worship Jesus Christ, who created us and recreated us.

Christians who meet together on Sunday to worship the Lord are challenged to worship individually every day of the week as an important part of life. Contrary to the Bible, the pagan Greeks divided life into secular and sacred compartments. This attitude is prevalent today. However, Paul stressed that life is totally sacred and should be accompanied with worship:

> So whether you eat or drink or whatever you do, do it all for the glory of God. (1 Corinthians 10:31)

A joyful heart has medicinal value

Worship mirrors a joyful heart, which has

medicinal value. Medical science is discovering what was recorded in the book of Proverbs more than 2,500 years ago:

> A cheerful heart is good medicine,
>   but a crushed spirit dries up the bones.
>   (Proverbs 17:22)

"New discoveries linking the brain to the immune system suggest that [our] state of mind affects us right down to our cells," reported *Newsweek* magazine.[4] As we noted in chapter 1, the Pittsburgh Cancer Institute concluded that "joy—meaning mental resilience and vigor" was the second most important element in predicting how long patients with recurring breast cancer would survive.

Serious researchers are looking into what they call "grieving cells." These researchers say: "It is almost as if the body were turned inside out and the cells themselves were experiencing grief or fear or hope."[5] In cases of sadness over the loss of someone close, "the body grieves, too. Rates of illness and death tend to be higher among those who have recently lost a spouse."[6]

But the public appears to be doubtful about the state of the mind affecting them down to their cells.

> People may not be surprised that they blush when they are embarrassed, that a

frightening thought can set their hearts racing or a sudden piece of bad news can throw all their systems temporarily out of whack. Yet they find it hard to believe that mental abstractions like loneliness or sadness can also, somehow, have an impact on their bodies.[7]

Studies show that close relationships go together with good health and that loneliness has the opposite effect. These studies are proving what Proverbs 17:22 has taught all along: that joy has healing value. If you want to help a person with cancer, remember that being a cheerful friend will help to take away loneliness and assist in the healing process. A worshipful and joyful attitude on your part will be felt and appreciated.

Sadness about having cancer or losing a loved one needs to be expressed openly if the patient is to find release and inner healing. Christians who suppress their emotions over a long period of time and withdraw into shells of loneliness dishonor the Lord and open their bodies to disease. If the "grieving cells" studies prove to be true, then a "cheerful heart" produces "good medicine" that has healing value to the body. Likewise, a "crushed spirit" produces so-called "grieving cells" that "[dry] up the bones."

Proverbs 17:22 is telling us that three things happen to people who have lost their ability to enjoy life:

1. Joy is replaced by sadness and depression—a "crushed spirit."

2. The crushed spirit prevents healing.

3. This unhealthy emotional condition eventually produces an unhealthy effect on the body—it "dries up the bones."

For inner strength: the joy of the Lord

Nehemiah said to the gathered Israelites recently returned from exile, "Do not grieve, for the joy of the Lord is your strength" (Nehemiah 8:10c). The people had just heard the sacred Scriptures read to them by Ezra, and they were grieving over the waywardness of their forebears and the consequences of that waywardness. Nehemiah's exhortation is good for us, too. A lifestyle of grieving is unhealthy for our whole being. Rather, we should choose the joy of the Lord as our strength. Certainly for the person going through a program of repeated chemotherapy and bombarded by negative emotions, this choice is essential.

In my case, these destructive emotions and physical feelings of nausea automatically occurred on the days when I had my chemotherapy treatments. They also occurred as flashbacks triggered by certain familiar sights associated with the chemotherapy. My whole system had become programmed by the anxieties and nausea. I continued to experience all those same emotional and physical feelings even after the treatments were behind me. Adding to the problem, I feared the cancer would recur.

When I returned for my first examination following the final chemotherapy, the very sight of the hospital triggered nausea. The nausea became worse as I entered the building and inhaled the usual hospital odors. The wait for my examining doctor seemed an eternity. All of the old feelings burst upon me with such force that I wanted to run out of the hospital and never return.

Lord Jesus, I prayed, *how can I find relief to escape these dreaded feelings?* The Holy Spirit brought to my mind a verse from the prophet Isaiah that I had quoted many times throughout the cancer ordeal. Again, I quoted it over and over until it filled my mind:

> Do not fear, for I am with you;
> do not be dismayed, for I am your God.
> I will strengthen you and help you;
> I will uphold you with my righteous right
> hand. (Isaiah 41:10)

The power of the words began to ease the anxiety. To further reduce my stress, I walked up and down the hall several times, quietly singing several choruses and hymns of worship and praise. By the time the doctor finally appeared, I was nearly back to normal.

I commented about my feelings to Dr.

Miller. "I'm experiencing all of the same emotions just as if I still have cancer," I said to him.

"You will have to get that monkey off your back," he replied. "It's a common experience with cancer patients. One of my former patients, after the chemo treatments, was walking from his car to the supermarket when he chanced to see one of the nurses who had treated him at the hospital. Immediately, he was overwhelmed by nausea and upchucked."

The stressful hold of cancer does indeed cling like a monkey on the victim's back. It was true in my experience. The monkey first leaped on me when doctors gave me the traumatic diagnosis of cancer. It represented all of the destructive physical, mental, emotional and social suffering caused by the disease. Throughout the chemo treatments, the monkey strengthened its grip. The effects of "making you sick to make you well" gave the monkey added weight, to the point that it was nearly unbearable, both physically and emotionally.

After the treatments were completed and I was in a state of remission, I desperately tried to shake the monkey from my back, but without success. Finally, after six months or a year, it dropped off of its own accord. But it has left its claw marks in me as a vivid reminder of its former presence.

Four spiritual resources

All who have gone through the trauma of

living with cancer can identify with me and that wretched monkey. Even though I knew by faith that lymphoma was not terminal for me, nevertheless I experienced the reality of Dr. Miller's "monkey on my back." My faith was tested severely throughout all the treatments. I had to marshall all of the spiritual resources I could think of to do battle with the monkey. I promised the Lord that I would share these resources with others to raise their hope and faith as they coped with cancer.

As I look back on the entire experience, I followed a pattern that had specific ingredients:

1. *A support base.* I was not alone. My wife, Elaine, was by my side. She fulfilled her role as a faithful wife "in sickness and in health, till death do us part," as the wedding vow puts it. And Stephen and David, our sons, were supportive. Daily family devotions were an important part of that support. I also had the loving support of my church congregation, including their heartfelt prayers.

2. *Prayer.* I seemed to be talking to the Lord almost constantly, asking Him to carry me through. My life was literally a life of prayer. Sometimes I wondered if God was not tired of hearing me call out for help. Also, as I just mentioned, I had the prayer support of my church.

3. *A Bible-filled mind.* I meditated on and memorized verses of Scripture that promised strength and healing.

4. *A heart lifted in worship.* I worshiped the Lord Jesus both in personal words of praise and through the avenue of music and songs. I found myself often singing. I would get out my guitar and sing choruses and hymns as I strummed. Of course, since I am a pastor, I was also involved in active worship in the church I served.

These four spiritual resources made it possible for me to creatively cope with all the negative feelings that cancer hurled against me.

Worship is a test of wholeness

What produces the greatest positive, creative attitude, uniting spirit, soul and body in harmony with our Father in heaven? It is worship! When cancer patients, whether in treatment, remission or terminal, worship the Lord in spirit and in truth, they are affirming that the Holy Spirit has control of their total persons. Their hearts are in tune with God. A.W. Tozer tells how the Holy Spirit enables people to worship the Lord acceptably to bring about this harmonious unity:

> It is the operation of the Spirit of God within us that enables us to worship God acceptably through that person we call Jesus Christ, who is Himself God. So worship originates with God and comes back to us and is reflected from us, as a mirror. God accepts no other kind of worship.[8]

Luke, in his gospel, relates the story of 10 people suffering from leprosy who went to Jesus for healing. Jesus told them to go show themselves to the priest—the prescribed way under Jewish law of ascertaining their fitness to reenter society. Luke says:

> One of them, when he saw he was healed, came back, praising God in a loud voice. He threw himself at Jesus' feet and thanked him. . . .
> Jesus asked, "Were not all ten cleansed? Where are the other nine? . . ." Then he said to him, "Rise and go; your faith has made you well." (Luke 17:15–19)

We have the choice of two basic attitudes, mentioned in our second chapter: (1) We can choose to live self-centered lives and miss the joyful, thankful attitude of worship. (2) We can choose to live a Christ-centered life, letting our attitude mirror our worship of Jesus; this will bring glory to God in all of our life. We see these two attitudes in the lives of the 10 men with leprosy.

1. *Worship is the missing spiritual attitude in the self-centered person.* Jesus had compassion when He saw the 10 leprous men calling to Him from a distance, begging for mercy. They wanted physical healing from leprosy and its ugly deformities. Furthermore, the law of the day demanded segregation for anyone with

leprosy. These hopeless physical rejects longed for healing so they could return to society and live normal lives with their families and friends. In Jesus, whose reputation for healing miracles had spread throughout the country, they saw a way out of their hopelessness. Jesus, in compassion, healed all 10.

But rooted in nine of the 10 men was the problem of self-centeredness. Life for them existed only in the areas of their minds, bodies and social interests. The spiritual dimension was missing. They wanted healing from their disease as quickly as possible so they could take their places in society. Life did not rise to any higher level. They had no desire to be made truly whole. They missed their greatest opportunity to be healed spiritually. They missed the greater miracle of eternal life, which was of more value than their physical healing. The physical healing might lengthen their lives by a few years, but spiritual life is forever.

Doctors, nurses and patients today need to recognize that healing is more than prolonging life for a few more years, though I do not underestimate the value—and desirability—of extended life. Modern medicine, as we have seen, has the ability to prolong life. But it is Jesus Christ alone who can save us from cancerlike sin, who can cleanse us of all unrighteousness, who can heal us spiritually and give us the gift of eternal life. D. Martin Lloyd-Jones offers this challenge on wholeness to Christian doctors:

> Christian doctors, there is only one way in which we can really make men whole! Modern medicine has gained much for mankind and it may gain much more. But when it has done its utmost it can only prolong man's life for a few more years. It cannot do more than repair a man's mind and body. It has to leave him there. It has nothing to say to the most vital element in man's nature. At this point Christianity alone can step in. When it does so, however, it can impart to the man something of incomparable worth.[9]

When Jesus asked the tragic question of the one man who returned—"Where are the other nine?"—it indicated his disappointment at the self-centered attitude of the nine. There was not even a thank-you from this sizeable group. But that overwhelming nine-to-one ratio is sadly repeated yet today. How many of us who have been wonderfully healed, either through medical science or more directly by God's intervention, worship Jesus Christ for our healing? The nine men who did not return to thank Jesus are examples of the prevalent attitude yet today.

2. *Worship of Jesus is the spiritual attitude of a Christ-centered person.* One former leper was so

filled with thanksgiving for his healing that he returned and "praising God in a loud voice . . . threw himself at Jesus' feet and thanked him." He had come into a new and living relationship with Jesus, who had made him whole. His interest extended beyond the mental, physical and social to a spiritual relationship with the living Savior. He alone of them was made truly whole.

It is unfortunate that the majority of people are interested in physical healing alone. They live life on the physical level rather than on the spiritual. And, as the nine men in Jesus' day, they miss the opportunity to be made truly whole.

Worship will be our eternal occupation

In Revelation, worship occupies a large segment of chapters 4 and 5, with other references to worship throughout the rest of the book. Worship is a celebration that begins in this life and will continue throughout eternity. The apostle John was transported "in the Spirit" to the very throne of God, the supreme power center of the universe. What was remarkable to John upon his arrival was the celebration of worship that surrounded God's throne. Look with me at that future celebration and see the three essentials for a proper attitude of worship:

1. *Worship is a celebration of the Triune God's character.* John remarks of the scene:

> Day and night they never stop saying:
> "Holy, holy, holy
>   is the Lord God Almighty,
> who was, and is, and is to come."
> (Revelation 4:8b)

We worship God for who He is. That is the key to a proper attitude of worship. When we have a deep understanding of the very character of God Himself, as taught by the Scriptures, we will worship Him more fully. The more we know God, the more we will worship Him in the beauty of His majesty and holiness.

2. *Worship is a celebration of what God has created.* Worshiping God for what He does is the second key to a proper attitude of worship.

> You are worthy, our Lord and God,
>   to receive glory and honor and power,
> for you created all things,
>   and by your will they were created
>   and have their being. (Revelation 4:11)

The saints around God's throne praised Him for His threefold work of creation: (a) All things in the universe, (b) the universe itself and (c) man, the crowning achievement of God's creative work. When we give recognition to the God of creation, we have a reason to join the saints of all ages in the celebration of God's worth.

3. *Worship is a celebration of who we are*

through the Triune God. John witnessed the 24 heavenly elders singing "a new song":

> You are worthy to take the scroll
>   and to open its seals,
> because you were slain,
>   and with your blood you purchased men
>   for God
>   from every tribe and language and
>   people and nation.
> You have made them to be a kingdom and
>   priests to serve our God,
>   and they will reign on the earth.
>   (Revelation 5:9–10)

Worshiping God for who we are is the third key to a proper attitude of worship. "Who am I?" is one of our cries as human beings. The 24 elders, in their doxology, describe the identity of Christians.

First, Christians are related to Jesus, who purchased their salvation with His shed blood as the Lamb of God: "You were slain, and with your blood you purchased men for God."

Second, Christians are priests belonging to God's kingdom: "You have made them to be a kingdom and priests to serve our God."

Third, Christians are identified as those who will reign with Christ on the earth: "They will reign on the earth."

Worship begins now

This eternal celebration around the throne of God is centered on who God is, what He has done and who we are. And those three fathomless concepts should motivate us to worship God on earth—now. True worship is our active response to God and the Lamb of God to declare Their worth.

> Worthy is the Lamb, who was slain,
> to receive power and wealth and wisdom
>   and strength
> and honor and glory and praise!
>   (Revelation 5:12)

> To him who sits on the throne and to the
>   Lamb
> be praise and honor and glory and power,
>   for ever and ever! (5:13b)

Heart-Talk

Emotionally (I feel): I have mixed emotions. I'm glad the treatments have ended, but my whole system has become so programmed by the chemo that I'm having flashbacks. I'm also having many of the old negative emotions. I want to feel good again. I have a nagging fear that the cancer will return.

Intellectually (I think): I am meditating on these healing verses:

One thing I do: Forgetting what is behind and straining toward what is ahead, I press on toward the goal to win the prize for which God has called me heavenward in Christ Jesus. (Philippians 3:13b–14)

Let the peace of Christ rule in your hearts, since as members of one body you were called to peace. And be thankful. Let the word of Christ dwell in you richly as you teach and admonish one another with all wisdom, and as you sing psalms, hymns and spiritual songs with gratitude in your hearts to God. And whatever you do, whether in word or deed, do it all in the name of the Lord Jesus, giving thanks to God the Father through him. (Colossians 3:15–17)

After this I looked and there before me was a great multitude that no one could count, from every nation, tribe, people and language, standing before the throne and in front of the Lamb. They were wearing white robes and were holding palm branches in their hands. And they cried out in a loud voice:
"Salvation belongs to our God,
who sits on the throne,

and to the Lamb." (Revelation 7:9–10)

Volitionally (I choose): I choose to celebrate all of life that remains by worshiping Jesus. I will put behind me the negative emotions. I choose to replace the flashbacks with psalms, hymns and spiritual songs sung in my heart to God. I choose to set my heart on heaven and to join all saints with the eternal celebration of worship.

Prayer

Dear Heavenly Father, I thank You for helping me to learn that life is sacred and that worship of Jesus touches all of life. Forgive me for the times I have failed to experience Your joy in my life to share with others. I worship You for the many wonders of Your creation. Develop within me a childlike awe that will cause me to worship You in all aspects of my life. May every day be one of joyful celebration to prepare me for the eternal celebration around Your throne. In Jesus' name, amen.

Your Invitation to
an Eternal Celebration

Who: Every born-again believer
Where: The throne of God
When: At death—upon departure into heaven
Price: Purchased by the priceless blood of Jesus

See spectacular sights never equalled on earth.

See the very throne of God where every creative act of the universe was conceived and executed!

See the beauty of the rainbow, resembling an emerald, encircling the throne of God!

See spectacular flashes of lightning more fascinating than any laser show! Listen to the peals of thunder!

See not only your guardian angel but listen to a choir of millions of angels accompanied by millions of harps!

All of this spectacular display is just the beginning of the eternal celebration that is guaranteed to be the greatest spiritual, mental, emotional, physical and social celebration of all time!

But none of the above will compare with your first glimpse of Jesus standing in the center of the throne. That split-second look will be so overwhelming to your total being that you will fall down in reverence and join the millions of saints and angels in worship and celebration!

NOTES

CHAPTER 1

1. Vance Havner, *Moments of Decision* (Old Tappan, NJ: Fleming H. Revell Co., 1979), p. 7.

2. Lloyd John Ogilvie, *Making Stress Work for You* (Waco, TX: Word Books, 1985), p. 182.

3. H. Norman Wright, *Self-talk, Imagery, and Prayer in Counseling*, Vol. 3 (Waco, TX: Word Books, 1986), p. 59.

4. Sue MacDonald, "The Healing Mind," *The Cincinnati Enquirer*, November 6, 1988, Section F, p. 1.

5. Ibid.

6. F. Minirth et al, *The Healthy Christian Life* (Grand Rapids, MI: Baker Book House, 1988), p. 139.

7. Jerry Bridges, "Choosing To Trust," *Discipleship*, May 1, 1988, p. 8.

CHAPTER 2

1. A.W. Tozer, *The Divine Conquest* (Camp Hill, PA: Christian Publications, 1950), p. 98.

2. *Everything You Always Wanted to Know about Cancer But Were Afraid to Ask*, United Cancer Council, p. 4.

3. "Cancer increase foreseen," *The Cincinnati Post*, February 18, 1989, p. 1.

CHAPTER 3

1. A.W. Pink, *The Sovereignty of God* (Carlisle, PA: The Banner of Truth Trust, 1976), p. 130.

2. William C. Doughty, *Healing from Heaven* (South

Holland: The Christian and Missionary Alliance Church), p. 8.

3. Lawrence O. Richards, *Expository Dictionary of New Testament Words* (Grand Rapids, MI: Zondervan Bible Publishers, 1985), p. 296.

CHAPTER 4

1. Robert G. Witty, *Divine Healing* (Nashville, TN: Broadman Press, 1989), p. 155.

2. Alfred Smith, "Cheer Up Ye Saints of God," *Action Songs for Boys and Girls,* Vol. 2 (Grand Rapids, MI: Zondervan Publishing House, 1975), p. 33.

3. Amy Harwell, *When Your Friend Gets Cancer* (Wheaton, IL: Harold Shaw Publishers, 1987), p. xiii.

4. Keith M. Bailey, *The Children's Bread* (Harrisburg, PA: Christian Publications, 1977), p. 46.

5. Richard M. Sipley, *Understanding Divine Healing* (Camp Hill, PA: Christian Publications, 1990), p. 121. Chart used by permission.

CHAPTER 5

1. Hal Lindsey, *Combat Faith* (New York: Bantam Books, 1986), p. 21.

2. Sue McDonald, "Hot Rocks for the 80s," *The Cincinnati Enquirer.*

3. A.Z. Hall, "The Cross and Caduceus," *Christianity Today,* January 30, 1961, p. 7.

4. Bill Gothard, *Basic Presuppositions for Wise Medical Decisions* (Oak Brook, IL: Institute in Basic Youth Conflicts, 1986), p. 5.

5. Maurice R. Irvin, "The Highest Kind of Faith," *Alliance Life,* September 30, 1987, p. 31.

CHAPTER 6

1. Abigail Trafford, "Medicine's New Triumphs," *U.S. News and World Report,* November 11, 1985, p. 46.

2. Edwin Kiester, Jr., "The Next 50 Years: You Will Be Healthier and Live Longer to Brag About It," *Family Circle,* September 1, 1982, p. 52.

3. Ricki Lewis, "The Newest Cancer Weapon: Yourself," *Health,* July 1986, p. 56.

4. Martyn Lloyd Jones, *Healing and the Scriptures* (Nashville, TN: Oliver-Nelson Books, 1988), p. 158.

5. Rob Roy MacGregor, "The Inevitability of Death," *Christianity Today,* March 6, 1987, p. 24. Used by permission.

6. Ibid.

7. C. Everitt Koop, "The End Is Not the End," *Christianity Today,* March 6, 1987, p. 18. Used by permission.

8. Edith Schaeffer, "Till Death Do Us Part," *Christianity Today,* March 6, 1987, p. 20. Used by permission.

CHAPTER 7

1. Miles Stanford, *The Complete Green Letters* (Grand Rapids, MI: Zondervan Publishing House, 1983), p. 257.

2. Mary Beth Moster, *When the Doctor Says It's Cancer* (Wheaton, IL: Tyndale House Publishers, 1986), p. 31.

3. Stanford, p. 177.

4. Ibid., p. 256.

CHAPTER 8

1. Annie Johnson Flint, "He Giveth More," *The*

Treasury of Religious Verse (Westwood: Fleming H. Revell Co., 1962), p. 39.

2. Tim Hansel, *You Gotta Keep Dancin'* (Elgin, IL: David C. Cook Publishing Co., 1985), p. 96.

3. Chuck Colson, "My Cancer and the Good Health Gospel," *Christianity Today,* April 18, 1982, p. 56. Used by permission.

CHAPTER 9

1. Harold Kushner, *When Bad Things Happen to Good People* (New York: Schocken Books, 1981), p. 17.

2. Paul Lee Tan, *Encyclopedia of 7700 Illustrations* (Garland, TX: Assurance Publishers, 1984), p. 1513.

3. Paul E. Billheimer, *Don't Waste Your Sorrows* (Minneapolis, MN: Bethany House Publishers, 1977), p. 36.

CHAPTER 10

1. Robert G. Witty, p. 145.

2. S.I. McMillen, *None of These Diseases* (Old Tappan, NJ: Fleming H. Revell Co., 1984), p. 15.

3. Ibid., p. 21.

4. Ibid., p. 23.

5. Jane E. Brody, "Cancer Prevention As Vital As Its Cure," *The Cincinnati Enquirer,* April 15, 1984.

6. A.B. Simpson, *Wholly Sanctified* (Harrisburg, PA: Christian Publications, 1925), p. 74.

7. Kathleen Cahill, "Ancient Wisdom, Modern Remedy," *The Walking Magazine* (Boston: Raben/The Walking Magazine Partner, June/July 1988), p. 39.

8. Bill Gothard, *How the Analogy of Christ to Bread*

Gives Direction for Avoiding Diseases (Oak Brook, IL: Institute in Basic Youth Conflicts, 1986), p. 1.

9. Ibid., p. 3.

10. Ibid.

11. Jane Brody, "Fiber can shrink some polyps," *The Cincinnati Enquirer,* September 6, 1989, p. 1.

12. William Pollen, *Why People Smoke Cigarettes* (U.S. Department of Health and Human Service (PHS) 83-50195, 1984), p. 4.

13. John N. Wilford, "3 drinks a week linked to breast-cancer risk," *The Cincinnati Enquirer,* May 7, 1987, p. 1.

CHAPTER 11

1. Billy Graham, *Till Armageddon* (Waco, TX: Word Books, 1981), p. 200.

2. Ann Landers, Chicago *Tribune,* April 11, 1977.

3. Frederick Langbridge, *A Cluster of Quiet Talks,* Religious Tract Society.

CHAPTER 12

1. Robert E. Webber, *Worship Is a Verb* (Waco, TX: Word Books, 1985), p. 33.

2. Ronald B. Allen, *The Majesty of Man* (Portland, OR: Multnomah Press, 1984), p. 201.

3. A.W. Tozer, *Whatever Happened to Worship* (Camp Hill, PA: Christian Publications, 1985), p. 56.

4. David Gelman and Mary Hager, "Body and Soul," *Newsweek,* November 7, 1988, p. 88.

5. Ibid.

6. Ibid., p. 91.

7. Ibid., p. 88.

8. A.W. Tozer, p. 44.

9. D. Martyn Lloyd-Jones, p. 118.

BIBLIOGRAPHY

Allen, Ronald B. *The Majesty Of Man*. Portland, OR: Multnomah Press, 1984.

Bailey, Keith M. *The Children's Bread*. Harrisburg, PA: Christian Publications, 1977.

————. "A New Significance for the Doctrine of Healing in the Atonement." *His Dominion*, Vol. 13.

Barnes, Albert. *Barnes' Notes on the New Testament*. Grand Rapids, MI: Kregel Publications, 1962.

Billheimer, Paul E. *Don't Waste Your Sorrows*. Minneapolis, MN: Bethany House Publishers, 1977.

Brand, Paul and Yancey, Philip. *Fearfully and Wonderfully Made*. Grand Rapids, MI: Zondervan Publishing House, 1981.

Bridges, Jerry. "Choosing To Trust." *Discipleship*, May 1, 1988.

Brody, Jane E. "Cancer Prevention as Vital as Its Cure." *The Cincinnati Enquirer*, April 15, 1984.

Cahill, Kathleen. "Ancient Wisdom, Modern Remedy." *The Walking Magazine*, June/July 1988.

Cassel, Eric J. "The Nature of Suffering and the Goals of Medicine." *The New England Journal of Medicine*, March 18, 1982.

Colson, Chuck. "My Cancer and the Good Health Gospel." *Christianity Today*, April 18, 1982.

Crabb, Lawrence J. *Effective Biblical Counseling*. Grand Rapids, MI: Zondervan Publishing House, 1985.

Doughty, William C. *Healing From Heaven*. Printed by South Holland Christian and Missionary Alliance Church.

Everything You Always Wanted To Know About Cancer But Were Afraid To Ask. United Cancer Council.

Flint, Annie Johnson. "He Giveth More." *The Treasury of Religious Verse*. Old Tappan, NJ: Fleming H. Revell Co., 1962.

Gabor, Andrea. "Medicine's New Triumphs." *U.S. News and World Report*, November 11, 1985.

Gelman, David and Hager, Mary. "Body and Soul," *Newsweek*, November 7, 1988.

Gothard, Bill. *Basic Presuppositions for Wise Medical Decisions*. Oak Brook, IL: Institute in Basic Youth Conflicts, 1986.

———. *How the Analogy of Christ to Bread Gives Direction for Avoiding Diseases*. Oak Brook,

IL: Institute in Basic Youth Conflicts, 1986.

————. *The Secret of Success*. Oak Brook, IL: Institute in Basic Youth Conflicts, 1986.

Graham, Billy. *Till Armageddon*. Waco, TX: Word Books, 1985.

Guinness, Alma E. *The ABCs of the Human Body*. Pleasantville, NY: The Reader's Digest Association, 1987.

Habershon, Adar. *The Study of Miracles*. Grand Rapids, MI: Kregel Publications, 1975.

Hall, A.Z. "The Cross And Caduceus." *Christianity Today,* January 30, 1961.

Hansel, Tim. *You Gotta Keep Dancin'*. Elgin, IL: David C. Cook Publishers, 1985.

Harwell, Amy. *When Your Friend Gets Cancer*. Wheaton, IL: Harold Shaw Publishers, 1987.

Havner, Vance. *Moments of Decision*. Old Tappan, NJ: Fleming H. Revell Co., 1979.

Irvin, Maurice R. "The Highest Kind of Faith." *Alliance Life,* September 30, 1987.

Johnson, Judi and Klein, Linda. *I Can Cope*. Minneapolis, MN: DCI Publishing, 1988.

Kiester, Edwin Jr. "The Next 50 Years." *Family Circle*, September 1, 1982.

Koop, C. Everitt. "The End Is Not The End," *Christianity Today,* March 6, 1987.

Koop, Ruth L. *Encounter with Terminal Illness.* Grand Rapids, MI: Zondervan Publishing House, 1980.

Kushner, Harold. *When Bad Things Happen to Good People.* New York: Schocken Books, 1981.

Lewis, Ricki. "The Newest Cancer Weapon: Yourself." *Health,* July 1986.

Lindsey, Hal. *Combat Faith.* New York: Bantam Books, 1986.

Lloyd-Jones, D. Martyn. *Healing and the Scriptures.* Nashville, TN: Thomas Nelson Publishers, 1988.

MacGregor, Rob R. "The Inevitability of Death," *Christianity Today,* March 6, 1987.

MacDonald, Sue. "The Healing Mind," *The Cincinnati Enquirer,* November 6, 1988.

Martin, Bernard. *The Healing Ministry in the Church.* Richmond: John Knox Press, 1960.

McMillen, S.I. *None of These Diseases.* Old Tappan, NJ: Fleming H. Revell Co., 1984.

Minirth F. et al. *The Healthy Christian Life.* Grand Rapids, MI: Baker Book House, 1988.

Moster, Mary B. *Living With Cancer.* Wheaton, IL: Tyndale House Publishers, 1985.

———. *When the Doctor Says It's Cancer.* Wheaton, IL: Tyndale House Publishers, 1986.

Ogilvie, Lloyd J. *Making Stress Work for You.* Waco, TX: Word Books, 1985.

Packo, John E. *Find and Use Your Spiritual Gifts.* Camp Hill, PA: Christian Publications, 1986.

Pierson, Arthur T. *In Christ Jesus.* Chicago: Moody Press, 1974.

Pink, A.W. *The Sovereignity of God.* Carlisle, PA: The Banner of Truth Trust, 1976.

Pollen, William. "Why People Smoke Cigarettes." U.S. Department of Health and Human Services, 1984.

Richards, Lawrence O. *The Believer's Guidebook.* Grand Rapids, MI: Zondervan Publishing House, 1983.

———. *Expository Dictionary of New Testament Words.* Grand Rapids, MI: Zondervan Publishing House, 1985.

Schaeffer, Edith. "Till Death Do Us Part." *Christianity Today,* March 6, 1987.

Simpson, A.B. *Wholly Sanctified.* Harrisburg, PA: Christian Publications, 1925.

Sipley, Richard M. *Understanding Divine Healing*. Wheaton, IL: Victor Books, 1986.

Smith, Alfred. "Cheer Up Ye Saints of God." *Action Songs for Boys and Girls*, Vol. 2. Grand Rapids, MI: Zondervan Publishing House, 1975.

Stanford, Miles J. *The Complete Green Letters*. Grand Rapids, MI: Zondervan Publishing House, 1983.

Tan, Paul Lee. *Encyclopedia of 7700 Illustrations*. Garland, TX: Assurance Publishers, 1984.

Tengbom, Mildred. *Why Waste Illness? Let God Use It for Growth*. Minneapolis, MN: Augsburg Fortress Publishers, 1984.

Trafford, Abigail et al. "Medicine's New Triumphs." *U.S. News and World Report,* November 11, 1985.

Tozer, A.W. *The Divine Conquest*. Camp Hill, PA: Christian Publications, 1950.

————. *Whatever Happened To Worship?* Camp Hill, PA: Christian Publications, 1985.

Verploegh, Harry. *Signposts*. Wheaton, IL: Victor Books, 1988.

Webber, Robert E. *Worship Is a Verb*. Waco, TX: Word Books, 1985.

Wilford, John N. "3 Drinks a Week Linked To

Breast-cancer Risk." *The Cincinnati Enquirer,* May 7, 1987.

White, Jerry and Mary. *The Christian in Mid Life.* Colorado Springs, CO: NavPress, 1980.

Wise, Robert L. *When There Is No Miracle.* Ventura, CA: Regal Books, 1986.

Witty, Robert G. *Divine Healing.* Nashville, TN: Broadman Press, 1989.

Wright, H. Norman. *How to Have a Creative Crisis.* Waco, TX: Word Books, 1986.

———. *Self-talk, Imagery, and Prayer in Counseling.* Waco, TX: Word Books, 1986.

Creative Choice #1

"I did not choose cancer, but I choose to trust God for courage to cope wtih cancer."

Creative Choice #2

"Cancer is a divine appointment to recieve Christ's miracle of His life into one's heart."

Creative Choice #3

"Since our soverign Lord permits cancer for His glory and our spiritual growth, I will glorify God and grow."

Have I not commanded you? Be strong and courageous. Do not be terrified; do not be discouraged, for the Lord your God will be with you wherever you go.
Joshua 1:9

And this is the testimony: God has given us eternal life, and this life is in his son. He who has the Son has life; he who does not have the Son of God does not have life.
1 John 5:11–12

"For I know the plans I have for you," declares the Lord, *"plans to prosper you and not to harm you, plans to give you hope and a future." Jeremiah 29:11*

Creative Choice #4

"Because Christ's death on the wondrous cross is the basis for divine healing, I choose His supernatural power to supplement my doctor's treatments."

Creative Choice #5

"I pick James's prescriptions administered by the elders of the local church, then leave the healing results to God."

Creative Choice #6

"If I select the wonders of modern medicine, I must be prepared to manage the not–so–wonderful side effects."

He himself bore our sins in his body on the tree, so that we might die to sins and live for righteousness; by his wounds you have been healed.
1 Peter 2:24

Is any one of you sick? He should call the elders of the church to pray over him and annoint him with oil in the name of the Lord. And the prayer offered in faith will make the sick person well; the Lord will raise him up. If he has sinned, he will be forgiven. Therefore confess your sins to each other and pray for each other so that you may be healed.
James 5:14–16a

On hearing this, Jesus said, "It is not the healthy who need a doctor, but the sick."
Matthew 9:12

Our dear friend Luke, the doctor, and Demas sent greetings.
Colossians 4:14

Creative Choice #7

"I practice positional thinking that produces power to live above tough circumstances."

Creative Choice #8

"When God withholds the miracle of instant healing, I humbly embrace His alternative of amazing grace that creates inner strength, and a joyful disposition."

Creative Choice #9

"I love God who specializes in the miracle of turning cancer into my ultimate good of Christlikeness."

And God raised us up with Christ and seated us with him in the heavenly realms in Christ Jesus.
Ephesians 2:6

But he said to me, "My grace is sufficient for you, for my power is made perfect in weakness. Therefore I will boast all the more gladly about my weaknesses, so that Christ's power may rest on me.
2 Corinthians 12:9

And we know that in all things God works for the good of those who love him, who have been called according to his purpose. For those God foreknew he also predestined to become conformed to the likeness of his Son.
Romans 8:28–29a

Creative Choice #10

"I dedicate my body to Christ and separate it from unhealthy eating habits, chemical abuse and overexposure to sun."

Creative Choice #11

"I accept death as the departure into heaven made possible by the resurrection of Jesus Christ from the dead."

Creative Choice #12

"I celebrate the wonder of life by filling my heart with the joy of worshiping Jesus."

I praise you because I am fearfully and wonderfully made; your works are wonderful, I know that full well.

Psalm 139:14

Don't you know that you yourselves are God's temple and that God's Spirit lives in you? If anyone destroys Gods temple, God will destroy him; for God's temple is sacred, and you are that temple.

1 Corinthians 3:16–17

Jesus said to her, "I am the resurrection and the life. He who believes in me will live, even though he dies; and whoever lives and believes in me will never die.

John 11:25–26a

A cheerful heart is good medicine, but a crushed spirit dries up the bones.

Proverbs 17:22

Do not grieve, for the joy of the Lord is your strength.

Nehemiah 8:10c

To him who sits on the throne and to the Lamb be praise and honor and glory and power, for ever and ever!

Revelation 5:13b